Ask Dr Ia
about
MEN'S HEALTH

DR IAN BANKS

Cartoons by James Campbell
Diagrams by Mark Hamilton

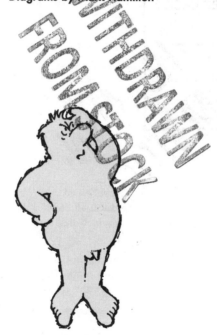

THE
BLACKSTAFF
PRESS

BELFAST

AUTHOR'S ACKNOWLEDGEMENTS

My thanks go to the staff of the Belfast City Hospital casualty
department (Maureen Turtle would have laughed in all
the right places); the *Belfast Telegraph*, especially
Jane Bell; *Men's Health* magazine, especially Phil
Hilton and Stuart Watt; the people of Blackstaff
Press, who restored my faith in publishers; and
my mum and dad, who kept me up to date.

First published in 1997 by
The Blackstaff Press Limited
3 Galway Park, Dundonald, Belfast BT16 0AN, Northern Ireland

© Text, Ian Banks, 1997
© Cartoons, James Campbell, 1997
© Diagrams, Mark Hamilton, 1997
All rights reserved

Typeset by Techniset Typesetters, Newton-le-Willows, Merseyside

Printed in England by Biddles Limited

A CIP catalogue record for this book
is available from the British Library

ISBN 0-85640-592-2

To Hilary,
who has suffered from
Men's Health for a long time

Contents

Preface

Men are starting to wake up to the fact that things could be better, much better. Let's face it, when it comes to men's health, compared to women's, things couldn't be much worse. We die on average years earlier than women, and for just about every disease common to both sexes, men come off worse. It is only recently that men and women have begun to ask why. Magazines and conferences dedicated to the health of men, and television programmes on men's health issues are appearing from nowhere. Unfortunately most of the information is presented in a patronising, as-from-on-high manner, often devoid of humour. Dr Ian informs without preaching. He gives the facts and, more importantly, suggests ways of changing the odds. He does not say that you must do anything, but, like horse racing, he gives tips about coming out on top. Nobody said you can live for ever, but living longer and being able to enjoy yourself at the same time gives you the last laugh. This book gives you the first one as well.

Being a man is a risky business

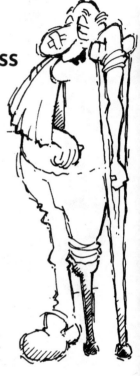

Men are a risky proposition. Many will be seen in hospital accident and emergency departments for various reasons and in different states of disrepair. Unfortunately some will never leave through the front door.

A 1994 MORI poll found that, compared to women, men had less understanding of the anatomy and function of their own bodies. Worse still, it was shown that women had a better understanding of the male body than men had themselves. Traditionally men have depended on women to look after their health and the poll showed that over 40 per cent of men will not attend their GP unless told to do so by their partner. In fact, 8 out of 10 men freely admitted to waiting too long before going to see their doctor. Now that really can be risky.

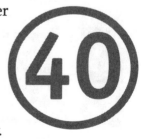

SPEED KILLS

Women, on the other hand, have a better track record. As well as looking after their menfolk, they seem to take much better care of themselves. For almost every condition common to both sexes men come off worst and on average men die five to six years earlier than women. So what on earth is it about men that produces these differences in health, illness and death?

Insurance premiums

Car accidents take the lives of over four times as many men as women. In fact, it is the single greatest cause of death in young men. This accident rate peaks between the ages of 18 and 25 years. Men in their forties have less than a third of the accidents of men half their age and most television advertisements promoting safer driving are directed towards young men. Some insurance companies now advertise special lower rates for women. Male accidents at work are also greater to around the same degree. Many industrial accidents often involve alcohol and protection, such as hard hats, is neglected or ignored.

Society has an ambivalent attitude towards men taking risks. Macho men feature prominently in the movies, and where would sport be without two men attempting to knock each other's head off, cheered on by a crowd often teetering on the edge of joining in? Boxing is perhaps an extreme example, but sporting injuries are common, particularly amongst men playing contact sports. In the so-called Oregon Experiment, the people of that American state were asked to prioritise those illnesses and conditions which they considered were the most deserving of treatment. 'Self-inflicted' injury,

(HIV infection came under this category) came very low on the list, while 'accidental' injury, such as sports injuries, rated much higher. Obviously one person's accident is another person's self-inflicted wound. Risk-taking has also been exploited by society. During the Second World War the relatively cheap fighter planes were flown by young unmarried men, while the expensive bombers invariably were crewed by older, often married, men.

End of the line

As the Samaritans will tell you, more than four times as many men take their own lives as women. After accidents, suicide is now the second biggest cause of young male death. It has increased by fifteenfold over the past decade and we don't really know why. While experts disagree on whether or not unemployment is directly involved, there is common ground over the benefits of female socialisation – women have a better social structure in which to discuss their worries. Men, on the other hand, find it difficult to admit their concerns, have increasing job insecurity and see once-safe promotions being taken by women. Their pent-up response can be just about as final as it could possibly be. Not only do men attempt suicide more often than women, they make a better job of it. Choosing hanging or car exhaust fumes to kill yourself leaves little room for manoeuvre. By favouring poisoning, women have a better chance of surviving a suicide attempt. If the suicidal man has access to a firearm, like soldiers or certain policemen, he will often use it to take his own life. Clearly there is little room for this method turning out to be a 'cry for help'.

Bottled up

For many men the solution comes out of the neck of a bottle. One in eight of all admissions to hospital from casualty departments are alcohol-related. Most of these are men. Alcoholism is on the rapid increase in the UK, yet it is declining in most of Europe. At the same time, addiction to

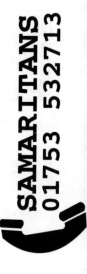
SAMARITANS 01753 532713

injected drugs is doubling every ten years, *but almost only amongst men*. Infections from injected drug abuse follow the same pattern, with men suffering increasingly from hepatitis and HIV.

Macho male

What has happened to us men? We need to drop the macho image, it hasn't really done us much good. More importantly, we need to find our new role as people equal in society and make sure the next generation doesn't fall into the same trap. Men make just as good parents as women. The big push is on to actually *be there* (as opposed to pushing up daisies) while our kids grow up. We don't have to be simply hole-in-the-wall cash dispensers.

Health risks

If you compare all the major killers, such as heart disease and lung cancer, men easily come out best, from the undertaker's point of view.

- Heart disease is the number one killer for men. One in three of us will die from either a myocardial infarction (heart attack) or a stroke. Worse still, one in six will die from heart disease before the age of 75 years. Testosterone may make us more susceptible to heart disease, while oestrogen may protect women from heart disease, but this is not the whole story.
- Lung cancer is the biggest cancer killer amongst men, a disease directly related to smoking.
- Cancer of the prostate will see off over 9,000 men each year in the UK, four times as many men than cervical cancer will kill women.
- Of the 130 deaths from testicular cancer from the 1,600 cases reported each year, almost none need ever have died.
- Even once relatively obscure conditions, such as melanoma, kill more men than women.

At the end of the day it is all down to the male brain, not to the Y chromosome. 'I would rather die young than be a 79-year-old cripple': this is the male brain talking. It has nothing to do with intelligence but a great deal to do with macho man. James Dean may have been immortalised on the silver screen but he is still dead. Better to be like Woody Allen: when asked how he would like to be immortalised, he replied, 'By living for ever'. It is the same machismo characteristic which leads to death from bowel cancer, testicular cancer and melanoma, not to mention heart disease and lung cancer. It is not that men are genetically more likely to catch something nasty, or even that they are less able to fight it. Having developed the lung cancer or heart disease from the life style we lead, we are less likely to attend our GP and when we do it will be much later than would a woman. It is mainly for this reason that as many men die from breast cancer as die from cancer of the testis.

Fortunately times are changing. There has been a dramatic increase in health awareness amongst men. In 1995 there were a number of major conferences and the launch of new magazines dedicated to men's health. Media attention has been intense, not least in the form of a Men's Health Season from the BBC.

Heart of the matter

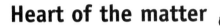

One of my patients complained that his legs were spoiling his sex life. Right enough his legs were on the short side, so I was about to prescribe a step ladder when he told me that he suffered from cramp whenever he performed exercise of any kind. I knew the feeling. Many an amorous night had been ruined by the 'pain with a mind of its own'. As cramp came on I knew that so much as a twiddle of the little toe would allow it to burst into agonising pain with me hopping around the bedroom like a demented pogo stick. This man had my sympathy and my undivided attention.

Cramp is actually caused by a build up of lactic acid in the muscles. This particularly nasty acid is produced when there is insufficient blood flow to provide oxygen. Without this oxygen, muscles cannot continue to burn up sugar correctly and a demented pogo stick is the result. You can, in fact, develop cramp anywhere there is muscle. Pain in your thigh which comes on particularly with walking is called *claudication*. It is caused by the arteries in the leg becoming constricted. Atherosclerosis is the main culprit and is a build up of fatty deposits, cholesterol and calcium, in the walls of arteries. This can happen in any artery in the body with often catastrophic results.

No one has yet designed a pump which will continue to work, at 2.5 billion cycles, without maintenance, for 70 years. The fact that the human heart will often do so, despite all the abuse thrown at it, tells us how far we have to go to match its performance. The vessels which conduct blood around the heart and body are also remarkable. Unfortunately it is possible to damage the heart beyond repair. Heart and vascular disease used to be so uncommon before the Second World War that doctors had to notify the coroner of a death from heart attack. Now more than a third

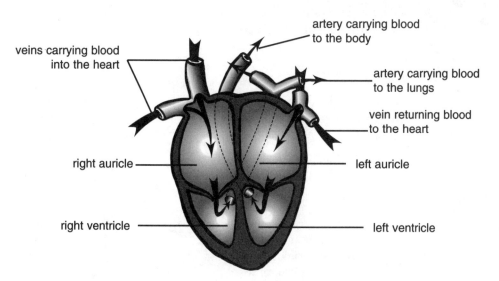

of all men dying prematurely, between the ages of 45 and 65 years, will die from a heart attack. It all boils down to blockage of the blood vessels.

Heart of the matter

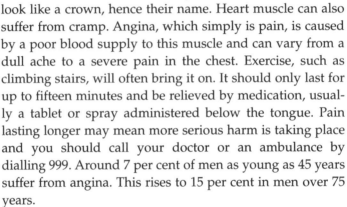

A human heart is about the size of a closed fist. It sits behind the lower part of the breastbone, more to the left of the midline than to the right. It is roughly conical in shape, reaching down to about the fifth or sixth ribs. The heart has its own blood supply from its coronary arteries. If you were to invert the vessels they would look like a crown, hence their name. Heart muscle can also suffer from cramp. Angina, which simply is pain, is caused by a poor blood supply to this muscle and can vary from a dull ache to a severe pain in the chest. Exercise, such as climbing stairs, will often bring it on. It should only last for up to fifteen minutes and be relieved by medication, usually a tablet or spray administered below the tongue. Pain lasting longer may mean more serious harm is taking place and you should call your doctor or an ambulance by dialling 999. Around 7 per cent of men as young as 45 years suffer from angina. This rises to 15 per cent in men over 75 years.

Men at risk

You stand a better than average chance of developing heart disease if:

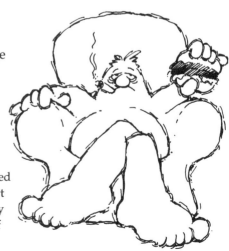

- You smoke. Smoking only 20 cigarettes per day doubles the risk of heart disease.
- Your father or brother died at an early age from heart disease. Thankfully many of the inherited causes of

heart disease can be treated but they are made much worse by the wrong diet or smoking.

- You have high blood pressure. We are still looking at the relationship between hypertension and heart disease but the two have some links.
- You have high cholesterol levels. This has to be taken in conjunction with all the other factors. These levels can be reduced and have been shown to be valuable in reducing the rate of heart attacks.
- You have a Western diet. Food rich in animal or saturated fats is a big factor, particularly if not balanced with whole food.
- You are older than 40 years. Risk of heart attacks increases up to 65 years then levels off a bit.
- You are white, Gujarati, Punjabi, or Bangladeshi, living in the UK. Your risk is 40 per cent higher than Afro-Caribbean men.
- You neglect exercise. A reduction of up to 50 per cent in risk is possible by regular exercise.

Detection

Your description of the pain will often give the major clue as to what is happening. There are some simple tests which will be performed, some by your own doctor but others in hospital as an outpatient.

- ECG (electrocardiogram). Much-loved by the television soaps, this examination can pick up electrical changes across the heart as it contracts. Strain or damage can often be seen as an alteration of the normal pattern. Computers now do most of the interpretation of these tests.
- Treadmill ECG (exercise ECG). A continuous ECG is taken while you exercise. For many men this is the first real exercise they have had for years, unfortunately often too late.

- 24-hour tape (ambulatory ECG monitoring). A small tape recorder rather like a personal stereo is carried around for 24 hours. It records a constant ECG of the heart which is then examined by a doctor or cardiac technician. It is particularly useful for picking up occasional changes in the way your heart behaves.
- Ultrasound (echocardiography). The function of the valves of the heart, in particular, can be visualised with ultrasound. Enlargement of the heart, and reasons for this, can also be assessed by this method.
- Angiography (cardiac catheterisation). Repeated x-rays are taken, following an injection of a small amount of radio-opaque dye into the heart blood vessels. This shows any constriction in the coronary arteries.

Treatment

Some drugs, such as nitrates, help open up the blood vessels, improving the blood supply to the heart muscle itself, and thus reduce the pain. Sometimes the vessels can be dilated by passing a fine tube into them and inflating a small balloon at the tip which is placed in the narrow section of the affected artery (coronary artery angioplasty). It has an initial success rate of over 90 per cent and can be repeated as necessary.

Really bad cases may need vessels grafted on as a bypass. This is referred to as a coronary artery bypass graft or CABG (pronounced 'cabbage'). A large vein is taken from the leg and grafted across the blocked section of the coronary artery. You may need three such grafts if all your main coronary arteries are affected. Only 11 per cent of people will still have angina after the operation. Most will return to work or their normal lives within three months.

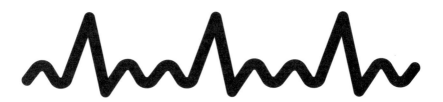

Attacks of the heart

Coronary thrombosis, myocardial infarction or heart attack – they are all the same thing and it is the single biggest cause of death in men. If the cardiac arteries become completely blocked, as happens in a heart attack, the pain can be severe and if the blood supply is not resumed quickly, heart muscle begins to die. This can seriously cramp your style. The heart can go into an irregular rhythm and eventually stop. If it is not restarted within three minutes, or if CPR (cardiopulmonary resuscitation) is not immediately given, there will be irreversible damage to the heart and brain.

How do you know it is happening?

Most men will know, and this can make things worse as adrenaline is released with fear which makes the heart work harder, thus producing more damage. In some cases, however, it can be put down to indigestion. This is even more dangerous, as it delays treatment. The symptoms include:

- A sudden severe crushing pain in the chest. It may radiate up to your neck, left or right arm or even down into your abdomen. Most men describe it as a 'tight band around their chest'.
- Profuse sweating.
- Shortness of breath.
- Nausea or vomiting or general feeling of being very unwell.

Ignore these symptoms at your peril. Over 25 per cent of men will die on the first day but most of the rest will survive thanks to early treatment.

Treatment

Always call an ambulance as well as your doctor. Many cardiac teams carry modern 'clot buster' drugs which can dissolve the blockage, preventing any further damage to heart muscle. Unfortunately they need to be used as soon as possible so don't delay in calling for help. If your heart stops, the team will restart it with an electrical shock provided by a defibrillator. Don't expect to wake up feeling like Sleeping Beauty. That guy drooling over you was giving you the kiss of life, not looking for bits of undigested apple. After the attack the heart replaces any damaged muscle with scar tissue. This is not muscle and will not contribute to the action of the heart. You may feel:

- Tiredness.
- Shortness of breath. The heart keeps the lungs free of fluid which will be impaired until it recovers completely.
- Chest pain, angina. This can be treated with drugs.
- Irregular heartbeats. Palpitations are common after a heart attack.

You will be followed up with tests to check on the recovery of your heart. Some drugs will help prevent a recurrence. Aspirin stops blood cells sticking together and cholesterol lowering drugs reduce the amount of harmful fat in the blood stream. Exercise is important and the last thing wanted is for you to be kept in bed.

Prevention

Despite the improvements in medicine too many men die from heart attacks. Prevention is the only real answer.

- Stop smoking. In 1994 the World Health Organisation showed that 50 per cent of smokers will die as a direct result of cigarettes. Smoking makes the blood clot more easily, promotes atherosclerosis, produces carbon monoxide which reduces the available oxygen, and destroys vitamin C which protects the heart. On the plus side, you might get free coupons for an ECG machine.
- Drink alcohol sensibly. This does not mean you should give up drinking altogether. In fact two glasses of red wine has been shown to have a protective effect. It contains antioxidants and prevents blood clotting too easily. Beware of exceeding the limit of 28 units per

week, as the protective effect soon disappears with
excessive drinking.

- Eat whole foods along with your fat. Simply
  reducing all fats, not just animal fats,
  does not seem to be the answer, the
  mix of foods is far more important.
- Eat more food rich in vitamins such
  as vitamins C, A, D and E.
- Reduce your salt intake. Remember
  most salt comes from processed food.
- Be active. It doesn't need to be the
  obsessive jog. Simply look for ways you
  can increase your activity. Take the stairs not
  the lift.

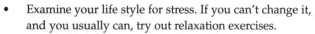

- Examine your life style for stress. If you can't change it,
  and you usually can, try out relaxation exercises.
- Reduce your weight if necessary.
- Take a good long hard look at sex. Some doctors believe
  a night's sex is equivalent to a five-mile jog. Mind you,
  hopping around like a demented pogo stick probably
  accounts for four and a half.

Other heart problems

Congenital heart defects include the so-called 'hole in the
heart'. Visions of a great hole in the heart leaking blood
come to mind but are far from the truth. Foetal connections
between the arterial and venous circulations remain open
after birth, allowing the mixing of the oxygenated and
deoxygenated blood. Surgical repair can often close these
'holes' keeping the two types of blood apart.

Rheumatic heart disease was formerly one of the most
serious types of heart disease of childhood and adolescence,
involving damage to the entire heart and its membranes. It
usually followed attacks of rheumatic fever. Widespread use
of antibiotics, effective against the streptococcal bacterium
that causes rheumatic fever, has greatly reduced the incidence of this condition. Even so, there are still people
around with heart murmurs caused by leaky valves
damaged by rheumatic fever. Artificial valves are one way

of helping if the damage is severe.

Heart transplants

In 1967 a human heart from one person was transplanted into the body of another. South African surgeon Christiaan Barnard performed the first such transplant; many surgeons adopted the procedure. Because most patients were dying soon after a transplant, however, the number of operations dropped from 100 in 1968 to 18 in 1970. The major problem was the body's natural tendency to reject tissues from another individual. Now heart transplantation is so common it is rarely even reported in the press any more. In 1984, in a controversial California operation, the transplantation of a baboon heart into a female infant was also attempted, but the heart was eventually rejected. A pig's heart – which can frankly be a pig of a job to find – may soon be seen as a suitable replacement for a human heart.

Artificial hearts

Artificial hearts have been under development since the 1950s. In 1966 Dr Michael De Bakey successfully implanted a booster pump for the first time as a temporary measure; at least one such pump continued to work for several years. The first permanent artificial heart, designed by Dr Robert Jarvik, was implanted in 1982 in a patient who lived for three months after the operation. A number of patients have received Jarvik heart implants and other artificial hearts since that time, but surviving recipients thus far have tended to suffer strokes and related problems.

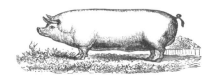

Blood pressure – the silent killer

It is not easy to recognise
that you have high blood
pressure without actually
measuring it. By the time
your nose starts to bleed or
blood appears in your urine
or your vision is only of any use
in the Channel Tunnel, your BP
has been elevated for a long time.
Headaches are not a good indicator, nor is a
big red nose. In fact, most men with high
blood pressure – hypertension – feel
remarkably well, like the calm before the
storm. Meanwhile, the heart is being
damaged, blood vessels in the brain are
under strain and the kidneys are suffering
badly. High blood pressure deserves its
name of the *Silent Killer*.

Pump up the pressure

Next time someone faints take a good look at their face. That horrible pallor and those rolling eyes are caused by the same thing – a lack of blood to the head. For a couple of seconds the pressure of blood leaving the heart dropped just low enough to prevent it getting far enough upwards to keep the brain awake. You will notice that people don't faint while they are lying down.

This is the basic flaw of any engineering design which has an oil pump lower than the crankcase. If the pump isn't working hard enough, kiss goodbye to your little ends. If the pressure rises too high you might find a trail behind the car not unlike that which followed the *Sea Empress*. You have blown an oil seal.

Humans have a low pump. Admittedly it could be inconvenient having your heart situated between your ears but it would solve a tricky problem. Every day the heart must keep the blood pressure high enough to supply oxygen and energy to the brain, yet low enough to prevent bursting a blood vessel. Exercise, sex and even just standing up require an increase in blood pressure. Strokes and aneurysms (a weak ballooning of an artery) result in a frightening number of people permanently failing their MOT. Unlike cars, it is not just a matter of taking the head off and having a look. Thankfully, strokes are decreasing as the relationship with high blood pressure is better understood.

Measure up

Measuring blood pressure actually involves two readings. The cuff wrapped around your upper arm or thigh is inflated to act as a tourniquet and the pressure within it is read off as a column of mercury forced upwards in a sphygmomanometer. As your doctor decreases the pressure in the cuff the heart is eventually able to force blood through the artery. This is heard as a sharp tapping noise through a stethoscope pressed over the artery on the far side of the cuff. You now know the *systolic* pressure corresponding to the heart's contraction. As the cuff pressure falls even further the noise suddenly softens and disappears. Your second reading at this point, the *diastolic* pressure, corresponds to the action of the arteries contracting. These are the top and bottom numbers of your BP.

Donor time

Not only do we have a low pump, it is not even a rotary design. After each contraction the heart must relax to refill ready for the next contraction. The brain cannot tolerate any stoppage of blood, even for a split second. Unconsciousness will result. To keep the blood shuffling along, the main arteries contract during this rest period. This diastolic pressure is not as great as the systolic pressure produced by the heart, but it is enough to stop you falling asleep after every heartbeat. Otherwise conversation, bad at the best of times, could take a severe turn for the worse, not to mention the performance of air traffic controllers. The diastolic pressure drops if the great arteries are unable to contract because of stiffness caused by atherosclerosis, hard deposits of fat in their walls. Fatty deposits also narrow the artery, restricting blood flow. Stiffness and reduced flow are interpreted by the stretch receptors as low blood pressure. To compensate, the heart cuts down on its rest periods and ups the pressure on each contraction. As a result, it works faster and harder with less rest, and the resulting high pressure can cause an artery blow-out in the brain. All this hard work with no rest also affects the heart.

Third opinion

As the arteries become harder, so the ratio between the two readings increases. At twenty years of age it should be around 120/70 mm of mercury, at fifty years this will rise to around 150/80. With severe atherosclerosis, pressures of 200/100 are not uncommon. The World Health Organisation defines hypertension as greater than 160/95, but age is a big factor. A minimum of three measuring sessions are required to give some indication of your average BP, as blood pressure varies dramatically. Just having your BP taken is enough to add 10 mm of mercury to your readings. Called the 'white coat effect', it occurs even if your doctor happens to be wearing a little black number. If your appointment was for 10 a.m., but you didn't get to see the doctor until 11 a.m., add 30 mm. When you go to see your doctor, get things in the right order. A rectal examination *before* your BP is taken will make that mercury column shoot up like a fairground machine. No free coconuts either.

Blood pressure is monitored in the body by stretch receptors in the artery walls. As the stretch decreases signals are sent to the brain, which then stimulates the heart's activity. Heart rate is not the only way of upping the pressure. By taking more blood in prior to each stroke, increased output will also raise BP.

Self-help

You can help keep down your BP without taking drugs. This makes sense as some anti-hypertension drugs can cause a number of side effects such as impotence, lethargy and depression. Even so, check with your doctor before stopping or reducing any medication, as a rapid rise in BP may occur and you still won't get much warning of trouble ahead.

Twenty ways to reduce your blood pressure

1   **Speak softly but carry a big stick**
    Anyone's BP can rise to near inner-tube bursting levels given sufficient aggro. Usually this falls just as rapidly and is referred to as a 'transient spike'. Do it often enough and you may find your BP steadily rising, weakening the fine vessels in the brain. Shouting ups the BP. Speaking quietly lowers your BP even if you are angry. Next time you are mugged, simply whisper, 'Go ahead punk, make my day, please.' You will still lose your wallet but you won't pop your top. Use the stick to hit yourself on the head for not buying traveller's cheques.

2   **Call for Dyno-rod**
    Straining at the toilet raises the intracerebral blood pressure. Feel the bulge on top of a baby's head when they are blue in the face from crying. It will be like a mole hill instead of a shallow depression. The same thing is happening to the blood vessels in your brain when you hold your breath against a forced exhalation.

3   **Carry a Bible**
    Lying is hard work. Not only do you need to desperately avoid giving the real version of events, you also have to make up a story of which the most eminent politician would be proud. Your heart rate goes up along with your BP and this is the basis of the polygraph for lie detection. Next time you are with your accountant, whip out the Bible and swear to God.

4   **Watch a party political broadcast**
Uproarious laughter stimulates the release of endorphins in the brain, reducing BP. Look for the best lines, such as, 'We promise to reduce taxes for everyone.' Regular laughter may permanently maintain a normal BP, so buy their video.

5   **Emulate Dr Who and get a K9**
Dogs lower BP. I'll rephrase that. Your *own* dog lowers your blood pressure. Other people's dogs can have the opposite effect, particularly while sniffing at your crotch as though you are hiding a sirloin steak in your boxer shorts. Pets generally reduce BP, possibly through relieving stress and triggering endorphin release. This protection diminishes rapidly with pet size. Polar bears give great hugs but only once.

6   **Get reincarnated as someone else**
Blood pressure is partly inherited along with your pattern of development in the womb. Fingerprints are formed late in the unborn baby. Bumps and whorls reflect poor circulation from the placenta which in turn reduces birth weight. Basically, the more whorls and loops you have in your fingertips, the greater the chance of hypertension. Men with at least one whorl have on average a BP which is 6 per cent higher than those with none. You will be relieved to hear that you cannot have more than ten whorls per fingertip.

7   **Lose your friends, eat loads of garlic**
Studies show that 300 mg (about three cloves) of garlic granules significantly reduces BP. On the down side, should you actually suffer a cardiac arrest, nobody will give you the kiss of life without first stuffing parsley into your mouth.

8   **Be a wino, in moderation**
    A couple of red wines per day, glasses not bottles, may
    well lower your BP. Recent evidence gives moderate
    alcohol consumption in any form the thumbs up. The
    protection is reversed with increased consumption
    beyond about two or three units per day.

9   **Take a tip**
    Caffeine from coffee or tea appears to quickly raise your
    BP. This immediate effect is blunted if you consume
    caffeine on a regular basis. There is now contradictory
    evidence over the link between
    heavy coffee-drinking and tea-
    drinking with heart disease. Tea
    also contains flavoniods which
    may have a protective value.

10 **Be Stan not Ollie**
    Carrying extra baggage
    around can get you into
    another fine mess. For every 9
    kg you are above your ideal
    weight, your diastolic
    pressure can rise by 3 mm of
    mercury. The good news? Weight
    reduction really does lower both
    systolic and diastolic pressures.

11 **Go for it hook, line and sinker**
    While the jury is still out over the effect
    on BP of certain essential fats such as eicosapentaenoic
    and docosahexaenoic acids, there is a direct link between
    the prevention of atherosclerosis and eating oily fish.
    You can lower your BP by simply not trying to
    pronounce these oils in the first place. Your fishmonger
    probably doesn't sell them by the pound, not filleted
    anyway. Mackerel is cheap and a good source of
    'healthy' oil, although those caught off Port Talbot at
    the moment may be more useful in your engine sump
    than in your arteries.

12 **Be of high morsel fibre**
    The World Health Organisation recommends eating at

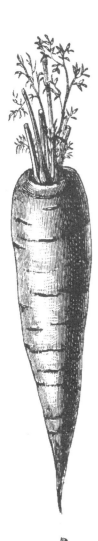

least half a kilo of fruit per day. Other natural sources of fibre are also excellent in reducing cholesterol levels. High fibre diets also help prevent transient spikes when you are sat in a small room with an echo and find your flat mate has used the last piece of toilet paper.

13 **Vegetate**
Antioxidants, such as vitamins A, C and E, help reduce the damage to your arteries by reducing cholesterol deposition. Go for carrots, broccoli, oranges and wheat germ.

14 **Don't shoot the albatross**
Drink at least two pints of unadulterated water per day to flush the kidneys. Hypertension can result from kidney malfunction with repeated dehydration.

15 **Have lots of sex, please**
The Olympic Committee decision that sex did not harm the world's athletes' performances, particularly the pole vault, probably depends upon when the event took place, given the medical evidence which favourably compares a good night's sex to a five-mile jog. However, sex most certainly does raise your blood pressure, albeit temporarily. Just thinking about it is enough to raise your BP by 50 per cent. If your cerebral blood vessels are badly dozed, this could be the last straw, if not rites. Even so, sex with a climax results in buckets of endorphins being released within the brain. BP falls rapidly, not unlike some other parts of the body.

16 **Develop a good stress sense**
Adrenaline is an ancient evolutionary hormone produced from small glands close to the kidneys. Heart rate and output both rise when the hormone stimulates the heart. BP rises and the blood is directed away from the gut and into the brain, muscle and sensory apparatus. You are now ready to either run away or fight. Unfortunately you probably happen to be looking at a computer visual display unit (VDU) showing your business slipping down the tubes and not a sabre tooth tiger drooling at the cave door. Chronic stress results in a gradual rise in baseline BP. On the other hand,

adrenaline is needed for top performance by actors and athletes. It is the 'burning off' effect which appears to prevent a permanent hike in blood pressure.

17 **Change sex**
Women suffer less from hypertension than men. Sex changes can be expensive, as hormones don't come cheap. On the plus side, your hair will return just in time for you to pull it all out by the roots.

18 **Don't be a salt of the earth**
Conflicting evidence abounds over the effects of salt on BP. It is becoming increasingly likely that other risk factors are exacerbated by a high salt intake. People with few such add-on extras are probably safer from the relatively high levels of salt we consume in the Western world. Some doctors believe that diets low in potassium and calcium are just as dangerous. Some fruits are loaded with potassium. Eat a banana and suck the chalk before you rub your billiard cue. It's particularly good for curved shots too.

19 **Fume if you must, but don't smoke**
Although they reduce stress, particularly during each budget announcement, cigarettes also damage the coronary blood vessels. This is exacerbated if you already have high BP. The only real way to protect yourself is to simply throw them away. There is as yet no medical evidence of hypertension in wheelie bins so feel environmentally free.

20 **Give this book to a friend**
Planning out what you intend to do raises your BP. Let someone else read the recommendations.

The last resort

When all the above have failed, your GP may advise anti-hypertension drugs. While not to be entered into lightly, there is increasing evidence that artificially lowering markedly elevated BP significantly lowers the incidence of strokes. It used to be thought that once you were started on drug therapy for hypertension you would be taking medication for the rest of your life. It is now well recognised that changes in life style, along with changes in diet, tobacco and alcohol consumption, can be as important as any drug therapy. Closely related studies also recommend the lowering of significantly raised cholesterol levels, a factor in high blood pressure.

Beating the Silent Killer is something to shout about.

Worked to death – work and health

A patient once told me, in all seriousness, that he had developed an industrial illness called 'lethargy'. He even had a note from his doctor which said, 'This man suffers from severe lethargy.' He was quite right. When I asked him to nip round to x-ray to check for a broken finger he asked for a wheelchair.

Industrial diseases are common. As soon as we started to use machines, spray chemicals or intensively grow food, it was inevitable that someone would have to pay a price. Child chimney sweeps in the 'wonderful' Victorian era developed a particularly nasty cancer of the scrotum from contact with soot. Some diseases only come to light with hindsight. Little was known about the dangers of radio-activity when women were employed to paint the numerals on watches with luminescent paint. The reason why you could read the watch in the dark was because the paint glowed from radioactive decay. Unfortunately the workers used to lick the paint brush to make a fine point before painting. Cancer of the jaw was the inevitable result.

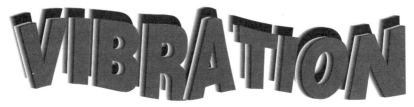

Industrial diseases still exist today, although control over working conditions is much stricter. Even so, legislation can be slow to catch up with medical research. The danger of asbestos causing asbestosis was known for a long time before workers were properly protected. Cancer of the bladder is related to certain sulphur compounds used to make rubber harder and more durable. Men working in such industries were more at risk. Using a vibrating tool can affect the peripheral nerves. Men working with jackhammers or other pneumatic tools need extended periods of rest to avoid the loss of power in their grip caused by chronic vibration. Loss of hearing is common among people working in excessively noisy surroundings. The use of a chain saw or tractor can permanently diminish your hearing. Really loud noise can damage your internal organs and is banned in Jericho.

Nurses and coalmen share a common condition of bad backs. Most of these injuries occur when the correct lifting position could not be used, such as a patient falling or a sack of coal shifting on the lorry. Painful backs are extremely common, particularly amongst honeymooners. This is caused by carrying too much luggage. Honest.

Nurses also suffer from a peculiar condition called 'mallet finger'. Rupturing the tendon which straightens the fingertips causes them to droop inwards. It is caused by bashing the finger against the bed frame when tucking in the sheets. When this happens to nurses they say, 'Goodness me. I appear to have a mallet finger again'. Or words to that effect.

VDU

Strain is common in men and just about every part of the body, including the brain, can suffer. A young male patient once told me he had a serious dose of VDU. I was about to prescribe a particular antibiotic accompanied by a paternal tut-tutting noise when he made himself clear. VDU may not be some exotic sexually transmitted disease, but it can still give you something to worry about. Working on a similar principle to television sets, the display is formed by a beam of electrons, fired from an electrostatic 'gun' hitting phosphorescent dots on the screen causing them to glow. The beam is tracked across the screen at speeds invisible to the human eye so that the separate pictures appear continuous. Coincidentally the eye works the same way. By constantly twitching the muscles which move the eye, the brain prevents fatigue of the cells in the retina at the back of the eye which senses light. If the eye is held completely still, vision gradually disappears. Watching a VDU for prolonged periods of time tires these muscles. Once they are unable to scan the light across fresh cells in the retina your vision goes 'out of focus'. This is exacerbated by fatigue in the small muscles which focus your vision within the eye itself. Resting your eyes by focusing on distant objects away from the screen every ten minutes or so will prevent this happening. So far there is no hard evidence of this causing permanent blindness.

Repetitive strain injury

Eyes are not the only things strained by working at a VDU. Constant work on a computer keyboard can cause a repetitive strain injury. Any continuous, stylised action, such as turning a screwdriver or typing, has the potential to cause tendon inflammation. Think of the ink tube inside a ballpoint pen and you will have the idea of how tendons are built. A thick sheath protects the tendon as it transmits pull from the muscles. With constant repetitive movements this sheath becomes inflamed, hot, tight and painful on movement. In severe cases movement is impossible. Muscle weakness then follows and gradually power is lost. Rest and exercise which avoids this constant motion helps prevent it in the first place. Finger and wrist exercises should be carried out every ten or fifteen minutes.

Brain strain

Brain strain can be more serious and even fatal. Boredom and tiredness are the biggest factors in causing industrial accidents. Over four times as many men as women are killed and injured at work. Most of these accidents occur on the day shifts, in the afternoon or early evening. Changing patterns of work are the best ways of avoiding brain strain. Strangely many men are hostile to change in their routine and feel threatened by it. 'You can't teach an old dog new tricks' is often the excuse. A sure sign that their brains are not being strained in the right way.

Hard to stomach – ulcers

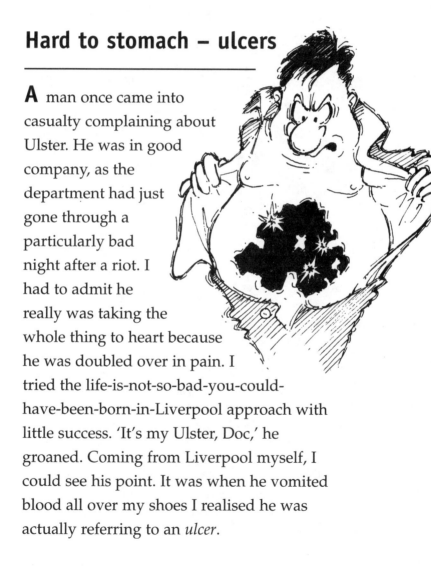

A man once came into casualty complaining about Ulster. He was in good company, as the department had just gone through a particularly bad night after a riot. I had to admit he really was taking the whole thing to heart because he was doubled over in pain. I tried the life-is-not-so-bad-you-could-have-been-born-in-Liverpool approach with little success. 'It's my Ulster, Doc,' he groaned. Coming from Liverpool myself, I could see his point. It was when he vomited blood all over my shoes I realised he was actually referring to an *ulcer*.

The digestive tract is a wonderful thing. It manages to eat meat without eating you too. Have you ever wondered how the stomach of a cannibal can digest other people but not themselves? It would be interesting to ask one someday, by telephone. The stomach produces acid which is as strong as that found in your car battery and enzymes to curdle milk which start the digestion of protein. This acid mix is then passed on into the duodenum, the first part of the small intestine, to finish the job. If the mucus lining of the duodenum breaks down and allows the enzymes to get at real meat, you have an ulcer.

Men only just outnumber women for all peptic ulcers, those which affect the stomach or duodenum. Gastric ulcers affect the lining of the stomach and are more common in men over 40 years. Chronic use of high doses of steroids, for asthma or rheumatic conditions, can cause a gastric ulcer. Even relatively small doses of anti-inflammatory drugs, such as ibuprofen or aspirin, can lead to an ulcer in the stomach in men who are susceptible. Duodenal ulcers are more common in men. They heal more easily than the gastric variety and usually develop just at the beginning of the duodenum.

Ulcers are common, with around one million people suffering in the UK each year. Of these up to 40,000 will need some form of treatment in hospital and sadly 5,000 people actually die each year. Despite better treatment, the number of people with ulcers has increased by 60 per cent over the past 10 years.

Symptoms

The symptoms of peptic ulcers tend to overlap but a fairly general pattern is recognised:

Gastric ulcers

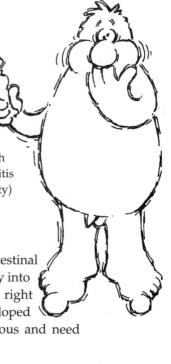

- Constant pain or cramps can occur which are particularly bad after eating (eating tends to settle pain in a duodenal ulcer).
- Antacids often settle the pain but it invariably returns.
- Belching is common, and embarrassing.
- Vomiting can occur.

Duodenal ulcers

- Most men know they have developed a duodenal ulcer at around 2 a.m., when they wake with a pain like a red hot poker just above the navel.
- Drinking milk can help but hot spicy foods make it much worse. Eating small amounts often relieves the pain.
- If the enzymes eat their way right through the wall of the intestine you have peritonitis (infection throughout the abdominal cavity) and a much bigger problem.

Emergencies

If your ulcer should erode through the intestinal wall into a blood vessel, you will bleed heavily into the gut. Worse still, if this erosion goes right through the intestinal wall, you have developed peritonitis. Both of these conditions are serious and need immediate surgery. Look for:

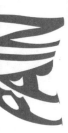

- Red blood or brown soil-like blood in your vomit.
- Black tar-like blood or fresh red blood in your faeces.
- Severe pain just below the rib cage.
- Dizziness when standing up.
- A strong thirst.

Risk factors

It used to be thought that only the jet set businessmen suffered from ulcers. Not so. It is more common in unemployed men. Stress is a major factor and can produce particularly serious flare-ups of the condition. Northern Ireland had a record number of ulcers during the past 25 years of violence. Tobacco-smoking has a direct effect on the ability of the stomach lining to produce its protective coat. This is not quite balanced by the calming effect most smokers feel they gain from their cigarettes. Over-the-counter drugs such as non-steroidal anti-inflammatory drugs (NSAIDS) can exacerbate any peptic ulcer and even cause bleeding in severe cases. This is made much worse by drinking any beverage which contains caffeine. Tea, often associated with calmness and sobriety, actually contains as much caffeine as coffee.

All in the family

Familial histories of ulcers are also important. If a close relative developed an ulcer, you have a higher chance of doing so as well. This is partly explained by blood groups which also run in families. If you are blood group O, you are not only popular with the Blood Transfusion Service, as your blood can be given to the largest number of people, you also have a 30 per cent greater chance of developing an ulcer than someone with any of the other blood groups. It's not all bad news. You may end up getting your own blood back again, as group O people tend to perforate their ulcers more often. It truly is an ill wind that blows no one any good. A factor that is equally important, however, is the area where you live, which will tend to be the same as your relatives. Men in the north of the UK suffer more from ulcers than men from the south.

Detection

From your history most doctors can give a reliable diagnosis. Unfortunately cancer of the stomach mimics an ulcer almost completely, so if you are over 40 years old, it makes sense to check it out before starting treatment. (Stomach cancer is very rare in men under the age of 45 years.)

- A physical examination involves prodding you in the abdomen. Ulcers have a nasty way of showing their irritation at being poked at and it will often be painful under examination. It makes sense to see if you are bleeding and a rectal examination is often performed particularly if you are in severe pain. Talk about adding insult to injury. Your doctor will also check for anaemia by looking for pale skin on the inside of your eyelids and palms of your hands, as some ulcers bleed very slowly.

- Now the real fun begins. By swallowing a radio-opaque substance, such as barium, the inside of your stomach and duodenum will light up under x-ray examination like the Blackpool illuminations. The big bulbs sticking out of the wall of your stomach are ulcers. It is called a barium meal, which gives some indication of doctors' humour rather than the standard of food in most hospitals at present.

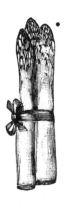

- Gastro-duodenoscopy is the definitive examination. It was invented by Japanese scientists to screen for stomach cancer, which is higher in Japan than in the UK. A flexible fibre optic telescope is passed into your stomach to look at the lining. Small pieces of anything suspicious can be removed and examined under a microscope. You don't have to do a course of sword swallowing to prepare for this test. Your throat is anaesthetised and you are blissfully sedated, dreaming of extremely long sticks of asparagus.

For the chop

Most ulcers will simply heal themselves. Stopping smoking will help. Eating small meals more often and avoiding those foods which cause problems makes a lot of sense. Avoid any aspirin-containing products – some of the popular 'stomach settlers' for the morning after actually contain aspirin. Check the label first; if in doubt just eat the label.

Surgical treatment used to involve cutting the nerves which stimulate the production of stomach acid and/or surgically removing part of the stomach which produces the acid. Thankfully these serious operations are now rarely performed, as powerful drugs such as ranitidine (Zantac) stop the stomach from producing acid in the first place. Antacids have always been popular and work by neutralising the acid produced. Most are simply chalk or bicarbonate of soda. Unfortunately long-term use of antacids makes the stomach produce more acid, so you end up taking even more antacids. Good news for the manufacturer; bad news for you. An excess of some antacids can cause problems for people with heart trouble and can interfere with medicines such as antibiotics. If you find you are having to take antacids very often and it is not really helping, check with your doctor.

Iron out the bugs

About 2 kg of bacteria share your gut with you. One type, *Helicobacter pylori,* is thought to cause stomach ulcers and possibly cancer; it is treated by antibiotics and a drug which makes the stomach work a bit harder by moving the food on through to the next part of the digestive system. Stress can also be a factor and simple relaxation techniques are often effective.

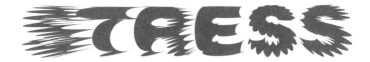

Deep in the bowels

Imagine the situation. You are alone in the lift as last night's main course of curried lentils makes an explosive escape at the fourth floor. Desperation turns to elation as the lift reaches your floor without stopping. The doors slowly open and in walks the entire typing pool. At the next office fancy-dress party you will be the only one not wearing a gas mask.

Along with excessive wind, the symptoms of irritable bowel syndrome (IBS) are intermittent constipation, diarrhoea and colicky abdominal pain. It affects one in twelve men in the UK.

Ten things you should know about irritable bowel syndrome

1 It affects three times as many women as men.
2 It is rarely, if ever, fatal. You only think you are going to die.
3 Symptoms can start at any age but predominate between 15 and 40 years.
4 Stress and life style are major factors.
5 The cause remains unknown.
6 IBS-associated diarrhoea is often worse in the first hours of waking.
7 Passing wind or faeces often relieves the symptoms.
8 Symptoms can mimic more serious diseases such as cancer so you should consult your doctor.
9 Diagnosis is based on exclusion of any other conditions. There is no definitive test for IBS.
10 There is no known cure. It is only possible to alleviate the symptoms.

Twenty ways to prevent or alleviate irritable bowel syndrome

1 Go for a high fibre diet containing whole grain bread and pasta. Around 25 per cent of men will find this actually makes things worse initially but it is worth persevering for a couple of weeks.

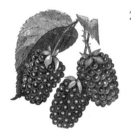

2 Eating plenty of fresh fruit can produce a remarkable long-term improvement in symptoms. If you can't be bothered eating fresh fruit, buy a juice extractor. You can use it for carrots, prunes and even bananas. Avoid commercially prepared fruit products as they often contain sorbitol, a sweetening agent. It causes diarrhoea in large doses, not to mention wind.

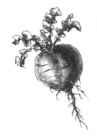

3 Dairy products can be the bad guys. Lactose intolerance is an oft-missed diagnosis. It is the main constituent of milk. Offensive, bulky stools, along with diarrhoea, can result. Try eliminating cheese, milk, chocolate, butter and

cream from your diet for a few weeks to see if there is any improvement.

4   Red meat, not just beef, can often send your bowel round the twist if you are prone to IBS. Aim for a trial period of white meat or simply cut meat out of your diet altogether.

5   Garnish your food with those herbs known to alleviate the symptoms of IBS – aniseed, chamomile, clove oil, black pepper, parsley and peppermint. You can also make herbal teas or infusions. They can be particularly effective when taken in the late evening, as many of the symptoms of IBS are worse at the start of the morning.

6   Stress can be a big factor, although it depends upon the type of stress you experience. 'Useful' stress comes from sport and activity generally. 'Useless' stress usually comes in the form of problems about which you can do nothing in the short term. Recognising useless stress for what it is is part of the answer to alleviating IBS. Don't forget, the bowel has receptors for the so-called stress hormones, such as adrenaline, which cause muscle spasm. Relaxation techniques really do work if you are prepared to give them a chance.

7   Active sex releases endorphins from the brain which counter the effects of stress. It also relieves a lot of pent-up emotion and frustration, both known to make IBS a great deal worse. This has to be the best excuse you are ever going to have and what an introduction at the next party: 'Together we can make beautiful, if basic, music.' Should knock 'em dead. However, some men with IBS find they suffer severe cramp in their large bowel just at the point of ejaculation.

8   Exercise is valuable. It increases bowel activity thus reducing bloating and distension. Almost any form of exercise will help but swimming is particularly effective. Avoid dehydration during activity, as this slows down the bowel and causes cramps. Eating a meal before strenuous exercise is unwise, as the blood is diverted away from the bowel when under physical stress; severe cramp is a common result, not just in those men suffering from IBS.

9   Nicotine stimulates receptors in the bowel, making IBS much worse. Quit the weed and avoid passive smoking. Most men with IBS symptoms report an improvement within three weeks of stopping smoking. Nicotine patches are designed to gradually reduce the amount of nicotine as the treatment progresses, so you can still use them to great effect.

10 Saturated fat not only affects your arteries, it also exacerbates IBS. Give olive-oil-based products a try instead of butter. Low fat fromage frais makes a welcome substitute for cream.

11 Sugar in whatever form tends to promote diarrhoea. Fructose is relatively easily digested yet can still cause problems. Diabetic foods, particularly sweets and chocolate, often contain large amounts of sorbitol which is difficult for the gut to absorb. It causes a profuse diarrhoea when eaten in excess. If you are diabetic and have IBS, consult your doctor. The good news is that many so-called 'diabetic foods' can be safely replaced with non-diabetic foods and can be significantly cheaper.

12 Bacteria live in the gut and are essential for the correct absorption of food. Eating live yoghurt can allow the colonisation of the bowel with *Lactobacillus acidophilus* which displaces less friendly fellow travellers. Relief from the symptoms of IBS for some men can be both dramatic and quick.

13 Burnt offerings can bring on particularly bad episodes of IBS. Avoid frying or roasting your food. Grilling, baking,

steaming or casseroling can help. Barbecues with plenty of oil poured all over the food are particularly well known to create problems. Eating the charcoal instead of the food can make more sense. (Please note: do not add more lighter fuel to the charcoal once you have started eating it. This can be very dangerous and will give you a bowel action Concorde would be proud of.)

14   Small amounts of alcohol can actually stimulate gentle bowel function. It is now well established that moderate intake of any alcohol, particularly red wine, can protect against heart disease. Some men, however, find that alcohol in any form irritates the bowel, making their symptoms of IBS much worse.

15   So-called aphrodisiacs like Spanish fly are notorious for causing bowel cramps and exacerbating the symptoms of IBS. Their mode of action involves the irritation of any mucous membrane which unfortunately includes the large bowel. Spanish fly also has a particularly irritating side effect called death.

16   Unadulterated water can be hard to find. The World Health Organisation recommends drinking a couple of litres of the stuff every day. It makes sense, but especially for men with IBS. Many cordials for instance contain additives which can make the symptoms of IBS worse. Better still, simply drinking plenty of water gives the body a chance to deal with all the toxins we consume on a daily basis. The large bowel is responsible for recovering water from the faeces but leaving behind all the nasty bits. It can do this far more effectively and with less damage to itself if there is plenty of water around in the first place.

17   Colonic irrigation is thought by some cultures to be the definitive answer to problems such as IBS, often considered a disease of the Western world. By passing a fine tube into the rectum and large bowel, a gentle stream of sterile water washes away any impacted faeces. While some people feel this is akin to having your tonsils

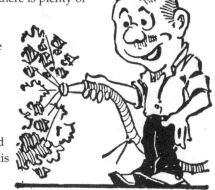

removed from the wrong end, advocates find it both invigorating and refreshing. Claims that it helps the IBS sufferer have some basis in fact, as slow movement of faeces is thought to be implicated in causing IBS. Even so, it makes sense to go to the experts. Practitioners in your area can be found by calling the International Colon Hydrotherapy Foundation in London (TEL 0171 289 7000).

18 Tea contains as much caffeine as coffee. Both stimulate bowel action which basically means diarrhoea in the susceptible male. Coffee also contains an unknown substance which causes bowel cramps. Cutting down on the number of cups of either tea or coffee makes sense.

19 Drugs are the last resort and have only temporary effect. Codeine relieves the spasm but can cause constipation. Peppermint oil is the basic ingredient of many drugs prescribed by your GP for IBS. Anti-diarrhoea drugs and laxatives work but long-term use of either is unwise. See your doctor if you constantly need to use them.

20 At the end of the day, and it usually is, the pain and discomfort of IBS can sometimes be relieved by a hot water bottle, or anything else which fits nice and snugly against your stomach.

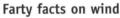

Farty facts on wind

Borborygmus is the medical term for the colicky pain and discomfort which accompanies a belly rumble; flatulence (wind) is the result. Sensors in the anal ring can to some extent detect whether pressure is being caused by faeces or wind. These are confused by diarrhoea often with surprising results.

Wind contains varying amounts of hydrogen sulphide produced from protein sulphide bonds broken during digestion. Protein from eggs and beans contain numerous sulphide bonds. It is smelly, poisonous to inhale, heavier than air and inflammable. Small amounts of air are swallowed during talking. This is either absorbed in the gut or passed as wind. Unfortunately passing wind also takes place while talking. With some politicians, only the smell helps you to tell the difference. Eating while stressed causes air to be swallowed. Muscle spasm causes a violent escape of this air as wind. Trying to force food down only makes it worse. Best to take a break and allow your jangled nerves to calm down. Doing a runner often solves the problem of who will pay the bill.

The only known death from wind is that of a patient on the operating table when surgeons accidentally ignited the inflammable gas in his bowel. Now doctors avoid using diathermy when performing such operations.

The *British National Formulary* is not impressed by drugs claimed to reduce wind. 'Activated dimethicone is of uncertain value,' it says. This is the main ingredient of Windcheater and Infacol. A wine bottle cork gives better temporary protection but invariably flavours the wine if reused. Some natural herbs reduce muscle spasm in the bowel preventing a build up of wind (see page 37, no. 5).

Hidden agenda

A patient arrived at the surgery and had not told the receptionist what was really troubling him. It transpired that he was bleeding from his anus when on the toilet. He also noticed that his motions tended to be loose and often very dark in colour. One of his brothers had died at the age of 60 from cancer of the bowel. When he came in to see me the first thing he said was, 'There is no way you are going to examine my backside.' Understandably I was a little confused because he was booked in with a sore ear.

One of the main reasons why men fail to attend their GP with problems of their bowels is the fear of a rectal examination. Some men will not even admit that they have a problem with their bowels and will appear before their doctor with a sore head or a cough. Only with gentle questioning does the real reason come out. This simple examination is the cause of a disproportionate amount of embarrassment which can be fatal. GPs perform it many times a week and it takes only a couple of minutes.

Labels on diagram: heart, lungs, stomach, liver, large bowel, small bowel, rectum, colon

Rectum? Nearly killed him

The rectum is the last part of the large bowel. Its job is to reabsorb all the water poured into the gut from the stomach onwards. It really can be abused by toxins hanging around too long, so it is best to keep things on the move as it were. Most cancers of the rectum will be within reach of a gloved finger making diagnosis relatively easy and early, so long as you attend your GP quick enough once you suspect something is wrong.

Symptoms

Watch out for any prolonged changes in your normal bowel habit.

- Diarrhoea or constipation which lasts for more than a couple of weeks.
- Blood or heavy mucus in the stool.

- A feeling of still wanting to go to the toilet after passing a motion.

These all need to be checked by your doctor. Weight loss is common but usually appears late in the course of the disease.

Risk

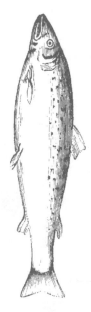

Cancer of the large bowel is the third most common cancer in men, and around 50 new cases per 100,000 men occur each year in the UK. More men than women die of bowel cancer, particularly over the age of 55 years. We are not certain what causes bowel cancer but we do know that your risk depends upon where you live, who you are and what you eat. It is relatively rare in Japan with its fish diet. Low residue foods are thought to cause a 'lazy bowel' which fails to clear itself properly – colonic washouts can remove impacted faeces. A previous history of ulcerative colitis (an inflammatory bowel disorder), bowel cancer in the family, or a relatively rare hereditary disorder called polyposis coli, which causes large numbers of wartlike growths on the inner lining of the bowel, all increase your risk.

High fibre, low risk

Fruit and raw or lightly cooked vegetables are thought to reduce the incidence of bowel cancer and the World Health Organisation recommends a minimum daily intake of half a kilo of fruit. Even so, early diagnosis usually results in successful treatment.

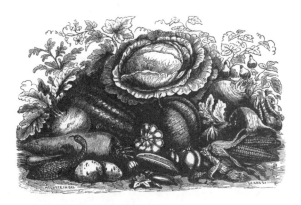

Treatment

You may be sent for a barium enema. During this procedure, air may be gently pumped in to inflate the bowel. You can make your own music as this makes its way back out. It is now possible to actually look inside the bowel and sample (or biopsy) any growths by means of a flexible telescope. Small growths, called polyps, are often removed during the examination and there may be no further treatment required. Radiotherapy may be used in conjunction with surgery. Larger tumours entail surgery, when the affected part of the bowel is removed. Sometimes the bowel is opened onto the abdomen wall for a few months to allow the rest of the bowel to recover. The bowel is then rejoined and works as normal. This is called a colostomy, and it may need to be permanent if there is no way of rejoining the two ends back together. Of all the people who are treated surgically for cancer of the large bowel, 50 per cent will survive for three years after the operation. Over 40 per cent will survive for ten years. Obviously the sooner the diagnosis is made the better the chance of a normal life.

Cough, please,
you've got a hernia

A patient once looked me
right between the eyes and told me
that he suspected he was
ruptured. I was in no
position to argue with
him at the time, as he
was sitting down and I
was on my feet, which
just happen to be
connected to very short
legs. 'Wot,' he said with
only the slightest change
of expression, 'are you
going to do about it?' As
luck would have it, my
examination with him in the standing
position meant I only had eye contact with
his chest tattoo extolling the virtues of a
homophobic life. Eager to please,

I managed to stutter that my wife had a tattoo just like his and I was seriously thinking of having all our twenty-five sons similarly adorned.

Generations of men have wondered why doctors hold their patient's scrotum or groin and say, 'Cough please.' The first thing that comes to mind is, 'Why are doctors' hands so *cold*?' A fleeting second thought that crosses many men's minds is, 'Why is my doctor smiling so much?' Most men, however, are desperately trying to avoid eye contact and are praying for their tackle not to respond in the way tackle is designed to respond when handled by another person. Car engines, the bank manager, even thoughts of Margaret Thatcher are all used as diversionary tactics to escape thinking about what is actually happening.

Not a laughing matter

This is a simple test, usually conducted in the standing position, and helps to detect an inguinal hernia. Also called a rupture, a loop of bowel or fat protrudes through a weak area of abdominal muscle. If the bowel has descended into the scrotum, your doctor will feel the impulse of the cough in the scrotum as the abdominal muscles contract. Sometimes it appears as a small lump in the groin, often disappearing when you are lying down or in the bath. Only when the bowel is nipped

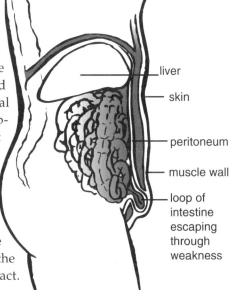

liver

skin

peritoneum

muscle wall

loop of intestine escaping through weakness

RIPPPPPP

and obstructed, 'strangulated', do you require emergency surgery. As recently as fifty years ago this was a common cause of death. Once the hernia has strangulated, the blood supply to the bowel is cut off and gangrene can set in very rapidly. Perforation of the bowel almost always occurs, leading to peritonitis (widespread infection within the abdomen). Thankfully death in this way is now quite uncommon but you should see your doctor immediately if your hernia becomes hot, painful or red, as it may have strangulated.

Strain pain

The abdominal wall is made up of overlapping sheets of muscle, rather like three ply laminated wood, flexible but very strong. The testes, which develop inside the body, have to pass through a small gap in the muscle just before birth. This unfortunately creates an area of potential weakness in the groin through which bowel or fat can protrude, and 20 per cent of those on NHS waiting lists are hernia patients.

Straining at the toilet, lifting incorrectly or even a violent sneeze can cause a rupture. You are more at risk if you are unfit or have recently undergone surgery. Surprisingly many men are totally unaware of their rupture. Some men will live quite happily with half of their intestines sitting next door to their testicles without coming to any harm. Others are only too aware of the event when it happens. One of my patients described a tearing sensation in his groin as he lifted out the spare wheel to replace a flat tyre. He now had two punctures. The fact that the spare tyre was also flat quite nicely took his mind off the pain. Generally speaking, the larger the hernia, the less likely it will strangulate.

Sportsman's hernia

Otherwise known as Gilmore's Groin, this hernia is often overlooked and patients, usually sportsmen, suffer prolonged and ineffectual physiotherapy for a presumed muscle injury. It is most common in sports that involve short sprints, abrupt halts and twisting actions, such as football and rugby. Most men suffering from Gilmore's Groin complain of a deep groin pain after activity. This eventually gets worse and is actually painful during activity itself. Coughing, sneezing and kicking a ball will often bring on the pain.

Cut and thrust

A truss, or surgical support, is basically a girdle with strategically placed pads designed to keep the bowel from sliding down your trouser leg. Over 4,000 per year are sold in the UK. Despite looking like a chastity belt, it can give a great deal of comfort and safety. Nevertheless, some doctors are concerned that trusses, when worn incorrectly, may make things worse by actually causing a strangulation of the bowel. Make sure you have the correct model for your type of hernia.

Surgery is the best answer. It takes less than half an hour and a couple of days in hospital after the operation. Keyhole surgery under a general anaesthetic reduces the amount of time spent in hospital but has yet to be fully accepted. It involves inflating the abdomen with a gas then performing the repair with the use of fibre optic telescopes. A revolutionary new method which uses a lattice mat instead of stitching to close the hernia has reduced the time in hospital to five hours. Advocates of this method say patients can return to work the next day and require no post-operative pain relief. At present that operation is not available on the NHS.

After any operation caution is the word. Gentle and progressive exercises to strengthen the muscle wall are essential to prevent a recurrence. Trampolining the day after the operation will show to everyone that you really do have guts.

Prevention is better than cold hands

Abdominal-wall exercises maintain muscle tone and help to prevent hernias occurring in the first place. If you are starting exercises after years of inactivity, use a firm support, such as strong Lycra shorts. 'Pumping iron' also pumps up the pressure inside the abdomen, so always wear protective supports. Some occupations which involve lifting require special training. Nurses are prone to bad backs and hernias. Pop stars are in danger of rupture from carrying their heavy wallets around all day.

Remember, anyone can develop a hernia. Some of the world's great statesmen have hernias. Gazza, on the other hand, has had two.

Did you know?

- Inguinal hernias are the most common to affect men.
- Women are ten times less likely to develop a hernia.
- In 1991 over 3.5 million working days were lost due to hernia repair.
- Bad news for us, seven out of eight sufferers are men.

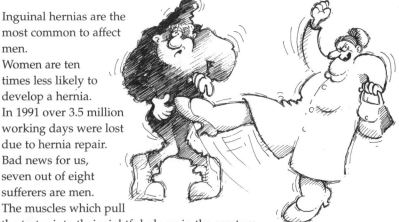

The muscles which pull the testes into their rightful places in the scrotum carry the delightful name of the gubernaculums.

Remember it. Threatening to kick a mugger right in the gubernaculums carries a certain weight of authority.

Get a grip of yourself

- Small hernias can be felt better if you stand up.
- Gently place two or three fingers midway along the crease of your groin above the thigh.
- Give a good cough.
- A gap in the muscle wall will be felt as a distinct tap on your fingertips. You may even see a small lump briefly appear at this spot.
- If there is obviously a loop of bowel sticking out, try gently pushing it back in. Lying on your back in warm water often helps.
- Ask your doctor for an examination.

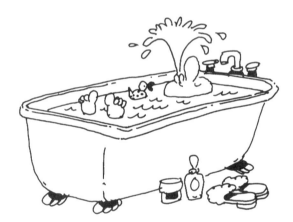

Medicines can seriously damage your health

Unless you happen to be a doctor or a pharmacist the prescription you just handed in at the chemist might as well have been part of the Dead Sea Scrolls. Chances are, the language used will not be so very different either. We are all encouraged to take our health more seriously yet it can be difficult to understand even the basics when it comes to taking medicines. To make matters worse, athletes, pilots and train drivers might find themselves on the wrong end of a hypodermic syringe to check for drugs commonly prescribed by their doctors.

Modern drugs are powerful. Unfortunately they can do more than just treat or cure. If taken the wrong way or combined with other drugs the result can be disastrous. There is information available, often on the medicine container itself, but in most cases it is in the form of an instruction rather than an explanation. Busy GPs may not find the time to make absolutely sure you know what you are doing when they send you out clutching your piece of paper. Yet it provides you with drugs which could seriously damage your health if the instructions are not followed carefully.

There is no such thing as a drug without side effects. Most of the time it is a case of balancing the desirable effects against the unwanted also-rans. New side effects are found every day, particularly for newer drugs. Doctors use a yellow card to alert the Committee for Safety in Medicines (CSM) of any possible dangers. If the committee gets enough of the same comments, it will, in turn, alert GPs and may even recommend a suspension of the drug licence. Tell your GP if you experience some strange effect after taking a particular medicine.

Drug companies are keen to sell their wares. Doctors are regularly visited by company representatives to explain the advantage of their products over others. Thankfully the days of expensive freebies are over but inducement and pressure can still be applied in different ways. EU legislation has brought the UK into line with the rest of Europe and pharmaceutical companies can only promote their drugs through balanced educational programmes.

A pill for every ill?

We consume several tons of medicines every year. Many of these drugs are not required and some will actually cause harm. It is worth talking to your doctor about their real value to you. Ailments such as coughs, flu and the common' cold are usually self-limiting in an otherwise healthy person and require no treatment. There is no evidence that they disappear any quicker with powerful drugs such as antibiotics. Doctors are kept up to date by the pharmaceutical industry and the Department of Health. The majority prescribe from a range of drugs that have been tried and tested and they know well. Most of the problems come from newer drugs prescribed by doctors unsure of their side effects. So, simply knowing what you are taking and how you can protect yourself from unwanted side effects could save your life. Always ask your doctor to write down what you need to know about your medicines.

Despite all the scares over drugs, medicine has changed our lives for ever. Infectious diseases were the greatest cause of death for children during the Industrial Revolution. With changes in housing, nutrition, vaccination and antibiotics, children now rarely die from such conditions as tuberculosis. Today we take painkillers for granted, but laudanum, a dubious mixture of heroin and gin, was once the only effective available analgesic.

Right medicine, wrong job

Innocently taking a medicine for your cough might make the difference between an Olympic Gold and writing your memoirs for *Life* magazine. You will still get the gold but not in a form you can hang around your neck. Read the medicines label carefully. Certain drugs can improve performance and are banned by the International Olympic Committee. Some common medical conditions can put you across the line when it comes to treatment. Driving while under the influence of drugs can invalidate your insurance. This includes any medicine which impairs your ability to drive safely. Some medicines produce drowsiness and you should check the label before taking them.

Generally speaking, the drugs which may improve performance are commonly used for asthma and hay fever. Medicines containing ephedrine (hay fever) or isoprenaline (asthma) are banned by the International Olympic Committee. Avoid drugs such as benzodiazepines (Valium) and antihistamines such as promethazine (Phenergan). Painkillers containing codeine can also cause drowsiness, particularly if mixed with alcohol. Never take anyone else's medicine and now is the time to clear all the old medicines out of your bathroom cabinet.

Read your own prescription

Doctors are now encouraged to use plain English when writing a prescription, and given the fact that most doctors need seven years to produce handwriting that is totally illegible, computers are a welcome advance. Even so, there are some popular abbreviations and Latin is still in common usage. Mistakes can be made, so it makes sense to know what instructions your doctor has written.

NP

Nomen proprium (proper name). If your GP crosses these letters out on the top of your prescription, the name of the drug will not appear on the label of the medicine. Yet all medicines should be kept in their original containers and you really need the name of the drug on there as well. Sportsmen should know what they are taking.

a.c.

Ante cibum (before food). Some drugs will not be absorbed properly when taken with a number 23 with extra bean sprouts. Take the medicine an hour before you phone your order. This should give you at least two hours before you actually eat anything.

p.c.

Post cibum (after food). This really means, take the medicine while your stomach is desperately trying to digest the banana fritter. Drugs like aspirin can cause gastritis when taken on an empty stomach.

o.d.

Omni die (once daily). Latin really does have a way with words.

b.d.

Bis die (twice daily). Now it starts to make sense. *Die* = day, see?

t.d.s.

Ter die sumendus (taken thrice daily). Shame, and just when you thought you had the hang of it.

q.d.s.

Quater die sumendus (taken four times daily). Generally speaking, the more often you need to take a drug the faster it is excreted or broken down. You can then make a good guess at how long it will be floating around in your blood stream.

stat.

Statim (take immediately). Usually written for an antidepressant after the pharmacist tells you the prescription cost.

p.r.n.

Pro re nata (when required). This is usually qualified by a warning not to take more than say, 6 in 12 hours. Worth taking note of, as it may only take 24 paracetamol tablets in half as many hours to kill you, horribly.

o.m.

Omni mane (in the morning). The body absorbs and responds to drugs differently at different times. Drugs causing drowsiness are often avoided in the morning.

o.n.

Omni nocte (at night). It sounds obvious, but the best time to take a sleeping tablet is at night. Unless you are on the night shift.

Warning: this medicine could seriously damage your health

WARNING: this medicine could seriously damage your health!

Labels on the medicine bottle or packet may include a warning. Combining alcohol with some drugs can be lethal. Even homeopathic and over-the-counter drugs can be dangerous when mixed with prescribed medicines. Cannabis, ecstasy, speed, and even poppers, can interact badly with drugs like antidepressants. Here are some common warnings and what they mean.

May cause drowsiness
Sleeping tablets, antidepressants, some painkillers and even certain antihistamines can help you drop off while driving on the motorway. Should be avoided when operating machinery or flying a Boeing 747. Particularly if I happen to be on board.

Avoid alcoholic drink
Some widely used antibiotics such as metronidazole will give you a nasty reaction to alcohol. Flushing and nausea are common but more serious reactions can occur. Alcohol and antidepressants really do not mix. Alcohol increases the effect of the drug, and has a similar and even lethal effect with sleeping tablets. Ask your pharmacist or doctor for advice if you are on any medicines and want to compete in the yard of ale.

Do not take milk, iron preparations or indigestion remedies at the same time of day as this medicine.

Calcium and iron bind onto antibiotics such as tetracyclines, commonly prescribed for chest infections, urine infections or acne. Many indigestion remedies are simply chalk, which is calcium carbonate.

Do not stop taking this medicine except on the advice of your doctor
Abruptly ceasing to take some antidepressants, antihypertension drugs or steroids can cause a rapid and uncontrollable return of the offending problem, along with disastrous changes in blood pressure. You should always seek the advice of your doctor before attempting to wean yourself off any such drug.

Complete the course

No reference to golf. Failing to kill all bacteria by not completing a course of antibiotics can lead to drug-resistant strains. We now have a strain of tuberculosis which is resistant to all known drugs for just exactly this reason.

Avoid skin exposure to direct sun or sun lamps

Some drugs prescribed for psychiatric conditions, and even certain antibiotics, can cause an overreaction to ultra-violet light. That healthy glow you develop after only ten minutes in the sun unfortunately disappears when all your skin falls off.

This medicine may colour the urine

Great one for public displays. Phenolphthalein is a common constituent of laxatives; it also gives you pink pee. Rifampicin is an antibiotic which turns your urine bright red. To really impress the troops, try the drug triamterine, used, as luck would have it, to increase the flow of urine. It causes a bright blue florescence when your urine is exposed to neon lights. Just the thing to brighten up any rave and makes such good reading in court the next day.

Takes more than a spoonful of sugar

Drugs are rarely given neat. They are usually mixed with other substances that increase or delay the rate of absorption, improve or worsen the taste, and create a distinctive colour. Called the 'formulation', it can make a big difference to just how the medicine is taken and whether you will bother completing the course. Drugs come in different formats; commonly used drugs which are swallowed come in three main forms.

Tablets

Solid and usually containing some inert substance simply to carry the drug or control its release. They may be coated to prevent being activated until in a particular part of the gut. Watch out for the abbreviations, e/c (enteric-coated), f/c (film-coated) or s/c (sugar-coated). The abbreviation c/c applies only to the doctor and means 'Crombie coated'. Coated tablets should not be broken before use. A score across the surface of a tablet allows you to halve the dose. A code, and sometimes a dose, is stamped on the surface to allow for identification. Peanut oil may be used, so if you are allergic to it, you should check with your pharmacist. Despite pressure from doctors, some pharmaceutical companies still make their tablets look like Smarties. Even more reason to keep your medicines away from little fingers.

Capsules

Gelatine is most commonly used for capsules. By varying the thickness of the gelatine, the drug can be delivered to a specific part of the gut. Stomach acid can render many drugs totally useless, so it is important to protect them until they have passed into the small bowel. If you break open the capsule to halve the dose, you may lose any effect from the drug. Sustained-release capsules contain the active drug wrapped in different amounts of inert compounds, giving a steady release of the drug throughout the day.

Mixtures

Good old-fashioned medicine comes in a bottle and is generally either green or red as people do not trust blue medicines. Children prefer syrups, although invariably most of the medicine ends up on you, or the floor, or the dog, which probably wasn't suffering from a cough anyway. Alcohol is a common additive and colours can include some of the dreaded E numbers. Check for: E102 Tartrazine; E142 Green S; E132 Indigo Carmine. Sugar is now less commonly used, particularly for children's preparations. That noise you can hear is Mary Poppins rotating in her urn.

Open wide please

There are much more fun ways of taking your medicine than just swallowing it. For some reason the French like to absorb their medicines by quite the opposite route and actively choose suppositories. As a doctor, I try to avoid ever saying 'open wide' to any Frenchman to whom I am about to give medicine. At least in the waiting room anyway. Americans like to spray their noses on the inside, while the increasing fad is for patches stuck to various parts of your anatomy.

Nasal sprays

Most popular route for decongestants. Successful trials with nasal insulin sprays may mean the end of daily injections for many diabetic people. Check the label for CFCs. Overuse only makes the problem worse once you try to stop. Nasal decongestants are great fun to use. Try it while in good company eating pea and ham soup.

Inhalers

Asthma sufferers will be familiar with the ubiquitous inhaler. The idea is to deliver tiny amounts of drug directly to the lung's many branching airways. This cuts down on the amount of drug required to relieve the condition. This can reduce side effects while administering the drug directly to the lungs, so allowing rapid onset of action of the drug. Carefully metered amounts are either sprayed under pressure, inhaled as a fine dust or spun into the air with a single inhalation. Theoretically many other drugs could be administered in this way.

Suppositories

The rectal lining readily absorbs drugs such as paracetamol. However, some drugs are not suitable for rectal administration. Aspirin, for instance, can cause intense irritation and even bleeding. It is best to stick to the directions on the packet. Rectal preparations are comfortably ovoid but bunjee jumping should be avoided for at least an hour after administration.

Dermal patches

Ideal for slow, continuous release, these patches are all the rage for hormone replacement, treating angina and weaning people off smoking. A new product containing testosterone is now available to replace the deficient male sex hormone in those men with measurable droop in this area. Dr Michael Carruthers of Harley Street feels that male sex hormone deficiency is more common than we think. He reckons the patch is an ideal way to make good the shortfall, if you follow my drift. As yet there is little scientific evidence to support his theories. A useful point to remember is that the hormone can be absorbed from any part of the body, bare skin permitting. You don't need to stick it where you think it will have the greatest effect.

With every breath you take

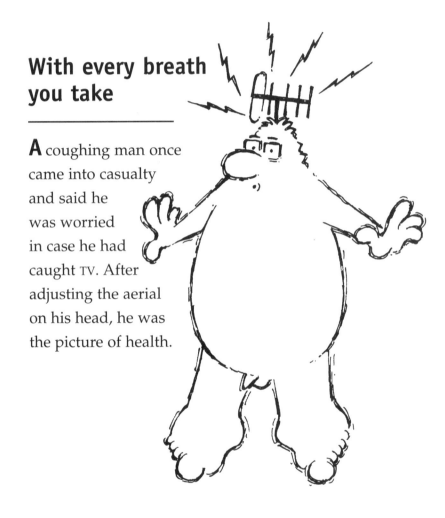

A coughing man once came into casualty and said he was worried in case he had caught TV. After adjusting the aerial on his head, he was the picture of health.

Lungs are not like plastic bags or balloons. If you imagine a pair of sponges connected to a vacuum cleaner hose, you won't be a million miles away from the truth. In the adult human, each lung is 25 cm to 30 cm (10 in to 12 in) long and roughly conical. They are covered by a protective membrane called the pleura. Infection of this membrane is called pleurisy. Nasty, and to be avoided. Inhaled air passes through the trachea, which divides into two tubes called bronchi; each bronchus leads to one lung. Air enters the lungs when the diaphragm, a strong muscle under the lungs, forcibly lowers and enlarges the chest cavity in which the lungs are suspended. This causes the lungs to expand, and air to fill the enlarged lungs. When the diaphragm relaxes, the lungs contract and the air is forced out. When you really need more air, such as when you have skipped the restaurant without paying and that footstep behind you is not an echo, the ribcage itself can also expand. A healthy adult can draw in about three to five litres of air at a single breath, but at rest only about 5 per cent of this volume is used. Vamping, that old Hollywood ploy used to entrap Humphrey Bogart, involved overuse of the ribcage muscles. I just thought you might like to know that.

Oxygen is passed through the thin membranes of the lung into the blood to bind to haemoglobin in red blood cells. Carbon dioxide goes in the opposite direction. Lungs have an efficient cleaning system to get rid of gunge that would otherwise build up in them. Tiny hairs called cilia waft the muck trapped in mucus up to the trachea, where it touches a sensitive area causing you to cough. Your sputum should be clear white. If you live in a city, it will be grey from pollution. If you have a chest infection it can turn green. A spotty brown and white sputum means you either have some blood in your lungs which can come from excessive coughing or you have inhaled a curried chip. Either way you need to see your doctor.

Diseases of the lungs

Asthma kills over 2,000 people per year. Breathing in is not the problem, it is trying to breath out which is affected. The small airways constrict on exhalation. This can be made worse by smoke, car fumes and even stress. The faeces from house mites living in the carpet, for instance, can have a powerful effect on the asthmatic lung and some vacuum cleaners will filter this out. Modern drugs help, but asthma is on the increase and we don't really know why. Perhaps if house mites could be toilet-trained a bit better, we wouldn't be in this mess.

Pneumonia can be caused either by viruses or by bacteria. Most people will fight it off and survive, and antibiotics can be life-saving. Immobility, caused by a chronic illness, will often lead to pneumonia in elderly people.

Asbestosis is caused by inhalation of asbestos dust. Many people died from this condition before it was accepted as an industrial disease. Dust from these workers' clothes also put their partners at risk. One man in Belfast developed asbestosis yet had no apparent contact with the substance. Only later was it found that the train he drove each day passed a ventilator blowing out asbestos-loaded fumes from a work yard. The asbestos had not affected his sense of humour. He told me he wanted to be cremated so he could be around a bit longer.

Tuberculosis was once a major killer. Most of the hospitals ringing Belfast, for example, were built only to treat TB. Thankfully improved housing and nutrition and, to a lesser extent, better medicine has reduced the risk. Even so, over 100 new cases of TB are found each year in Northern Ireland alone. Worse still, there are now strains of the bacterium causing the disease which are resistant to every known antibiotic.

Bronchitis is an inflammation of the bronchi. A constant cough and sputum is its signature tune, usually on the top deck of the bus. Shortness of breath is common and it is made much worse by smoking.

Mad, bad and dangerous to smoke

Lung cancer was rare until tobacco hit the scene. Sir Walter has a lot to answer for, but not nearly as much as the tobacco industry.

Tobacco-smoking in its various forms is the single biggest cause.

- The more cigarettes smoked and the younger the age at which smoking started, the greater the risk.

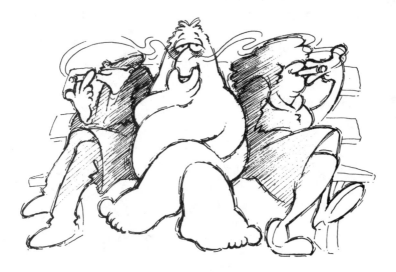

- Cigar-smokers and pipe-smokers have a lower chance of developing lung cancer, but their risk is still higher than for non-smokers.
- Inhalation of tobacco smoke by non-smokers – *passive smoking* – has also been shown to be a risk factor for lung cancer. A study in Japan showed clearly that the non-smoking wives of men who did smoke had a far higher level of smoking-related diseases than the non-smoking wives of men who did not smoke.

Lung cancer

Some things will not go away in a puff of smoke.

- Lung cancer is the commonest type of cancer in men, with over 100 new cases per 100,000 men diagnosed each year in the UK; 31 per cent of all deaths from any cancer are caused by cancer of the lung; 30,000 men develop it each year compared to 14,000 women, but women are catching up. More women than men smoke, most of them young women.
- The peak age for lung cancer is between 65 and 75 years; it is relatively rare in men below the age of 40.
- Few men survive lung cancer. Only 8 per cent will survive lung cancer compared to a 43 per cent survival rate in prostate cancer, the next most common cancer death.

What to watch out for

Most men will turn up at their doctor's surgery far too late to do anything about the cancer. You should go to your GP if you:

- Have a persistent cough.
- Are coughing up blood.
- Have an increasing shortness of breath.

Treatment

Although early treatment with surgery and chemotherapy can be successful, less than 8 per cent of men survive for five years or more after lung cancer has been diagnosed. Part of the reason for this low survival rate is the resistance that builds up to the effects of the drugs. It is unlikely that there will be any major breakthrough in the surgical treatment of lung cancer, but new methods of delivering the anti-cancer drugs are being developed.

Prevention

Giving up smoking, or better still, not starting in the first place, makes sense. Although radon gas, found in certain parts of the country, particularly around granite rock, accounts for 6 per cent of all lung cancers, smoking is responsible for most of the rest. Around 100 people die every day from lung cancer. Half of all heavy smokers will never reach 70 years of age. Even light smokers only have a 60 per cent chance of survival until the age of 70. Fortunately, the number of men in the UK who smoke is falling. There are now four times as many non-smokers as smokers, so you can do it if you try. Help is available:

- Nicotine patches can be obtained through private prescription. They can be very successful by easing the craving for nicotine.
- Get in touch with self-help groups or organisations which supply advice and information (see address for QUIT on page 199).
- If you can't do it for yourself, do it for your partner or your kids. Not only are they in the running for being one man down in the house, they can be affected by your smoke as well.

Things to look forward to after quitting

- Within 8 hours all of the poisonous carbon monoxide produced by smoking has been washed out of your blood. At the same time the oxygen levels return to normal.
- Within 24 hours your chances of a heart attack, much higher while smoking, begin to decrease.
- Within 48 hours the nerve endings destroyed by smoking begin to regrow. As smoking stops you coughing by killing off the nerves which control the cough reflex, you may well find yourself clearing your lungs better after two days smoke free. Your sense of smell will become stronger, as will your sense of taste. Many people put on weight after stopping smoking for just these reasons, they enjoy their food more.
- Within 3 days spasm of lung tissue decreases, mak-ing breathing easier. Lung capacity increases.
- Within 3 months your circulation has improved and you will have harder erections. Sperm count goes up, walking becomes easier and even your liver begins to improve (most of the detoxification of the nasties absorbed from smoke takes place in the liver).
- Within 5 years your risk of lung cancer has dropped dramatically, some doctors say by up to 50 per cent, and will return to normal within 10 years.

Easy to say, but . . .

Nothing is worse than listening to a non-smoker telling a smoker how to give up the weed. Nicotine is highly addictive and there will be withdrawal reactions. They can be severe and many men use this as an excuse for starting up again. Tension, aggression, irritability and difficulty in concentrating all get worse for a while. Not surprisingly 80 per cent of men will fail on their first attempt. You are dealing with a powerful habit as well as an addiction. If you smoke only 10 cigarettes per day this involves over 40,000 movements of your hand to your mouth in a year. No wonder men who are giving up smoking are always stuffing things, anything, into their mouths.

The Health Education Authority has devised a quit plan:

1   Set a day and date to stop. Tell all your friends and relatives, they will support you.
2   Like deep-sea diving, always take a buddy. Get someone to give up with you. You will reinforce each other's willpower.
3   Clear the house and your pockets of any packets, papers or matches.
4   One day at a time is better than leaving it open-ended.
5   Map out your progress on a chart or calendar. Keep the money saved in a separate container.
6   Chew on a carrot. Not only will it help you do something with your mouth and hands, it contains beta-carotene which inhibits cancer. Contrary to popular belief it will not help you see in the dark, until you forget what you are doing and try to light it.
7   Ask your friends not to smoke around you. People accept this far more readily than they used to do.

Changing times

A man turned up at his doctor's surgery. 'My dad used to tell me that during the war they were always told that cigarettes were good for you. Sort of calmed you down. Funny how things turn out sometimes,' he said. Not so funny. Especially if you are only 40 years old with three children and have just been diagnosed as having lung cancer.

Falling on deaf ears

I was puzzled the day I pressed the buzzer for the next patient and nobody turned up. Only after the third and prolonged attempt did a red-faced young man pop his head round the surgery door. He apologised for not hearing the buzzer, saying he must have dozed off. Yes, it might have been because of the long waiting times but not in his case. It transpired that he had recently attended a rock festival and had sat all day next to the speakers. 'You could really feel the bass hurting,' he told me. For the next few days he was almost completely deaf in both ears.

His hearing gradually returned but did not come back to normal.

We take our hearing very much for granted, yet men are notorious for failing to protect themselves from excessive noise which eventually causes deafness. Men are exposed to loud noise more often than women, but there can be few places more noisy than sitting in front of a bank of speakers at a rave. The volume of sound even from the tiny ear-phones of personal stereo sets can cause permanent hearing loss.

Party time

After being exposed to such loud noise at, say, a party rave, you may notice that your hearing has diminished. In most cases it will return, but with each exposure a gradual loss of hearing occurs. It can be hard to notice at first. You find yourself missing what someone has said, or, worse still, you hear them incorrectly. This can cause financial embarrass-ment when you rush to the bar after someone has told you, 'It's poor sound.'

The bells, the bells

Worse still, you can develop a constant ringing noise in one or both ears, which can literally drive you crazy. Many men will attend their doctors not so much because of a loss of hearing, which they presume will come back eventually, but because of the constant sound of bells, called tinnitus. It can also sound like a steam whistle, or wind constantly blowing, and is worse at night or in a quiet room.

Disco deafness

Loss of hearing caused by constant loud noise used to be called boilermaker's ear but is often now referred to as disco deafness. It is also known as the 'Do you come here often,

Pardon' syndrome. The fact that men lose their hearing more often, and to a greater degree, than women may reflect the macho dismissal of protection as effete. Working in a factory, with farm machinery or even with a chain saw can damage your hearing. The rave at the weekend, or the loud personal stereo on the way to work every morning, gives your ears little chance to recover.

Testing to destruction

Loud noises are prevented from reaching a sensitive receiving structure called the cochlea by a tiny muscle called stapedius. This muscle damps down the sound waves by contracting against one of the bones in the middle ear which conducts the sound. Acting rather like a damper or a shock absorber on a car, it allows only reasonable levels of sound to be sensed and transmitted to the brain. With constant loud noise it eventually weakens, letting the full force of vibration hit the cochlea. Continuous exposure to loud noise quite rapidly destroys this fragile mechanism and the loss of hearing it produces is invariably permanent. As it progresses you tend to turn up the volume on the personal stereo or sound system which only causes further damage. A truly vicious circle.

Deafness comes in two forms. Conductive deafness results from the sound vibrations being unable to pass along the middle ear bones, the ossicles, to stimulate the cochlea. Sensory deafness signals a destruction of either the cochlea itself or the auditory nerve which relays the sound to the brain.

Treatment

Conventional hearing aids don't always help, although a recent development of implanting an electronic device into the cochlea appears promising. Tinnitus is often impossible to treat effectively and some of the drugs used can also cause drowsiness. A constant, quiet noise produced by a small earphone from a personal stereo can have surprisingly good results.

Ear protectors, plugs and simply putting some distance between yourself and those speaker stacks makes good sense. Unless, that is, you want to spend your life nodding and smiling during conversation round a table. Get plugged in, pump up the protection.

Deafness can be catching

Ear infections are common but, thankfully, rarely cause permanent deafness. *Otitis externa* means inflammation of the outer ear. Fungus can grow quite happily in this nice, warm, damp hole. Small cracks form in the ear canal which can be painful and itchy. The natural response is to poke at it, which only makes everything worse. Drops can be bought from your pharmacist to stop the rot.

I once told a man he had acute otitis media, an infection of the middle ear. Quick as a flash he replied, 'I'll bet you flatter all your patients over their best features.' As I usually tell the jokes in casualty, I wrote him up for a tetanus jab just in case he slipped on the way out. Infection of the middle ear can be painful. The tube which connects the throat to the ear, the Eustachian tube, becomes blocked and so the eardrum cannot move freely. Dull hearing with a constant pain is the result. Like a boil under the skin, the pain subsides as soon as the pressure is released. The only way out for the pus is through the eardrum. Most people know that their eardrum has perforated when a smelly discharge pours out of their ear but the pain subsides almost immediately. Most of these infections actually clear up themselves but can be helped along with antibiotics. Mastoiditis, a complication which can lead to deafness and even brain abscess, is now rarely ever seen.

Superglue ear

A worried parent once phoned the casualty department about his child. I was able to make out the words glue and ear, so I recommended him to take the child to his GP. A few minutes later an irate dad turned up with his daughter. She had one finger stuck in her ear hole. It transpired she had been using superglue and scratched her ear with a goodly dollop of glue on her finger. This was not the glue ear we all know and love. Much controversy surrounds glue ear. Not only are we unsure of what causes it, treatment varies between doctors as well. To release the suction pressure which causes the reduction in hearing, vents, 'grommets', are inserted through the eardrum. This restores hearing but has its own small risk of complications, not least from the general anaesthetic required for surgery. Perhaps the best reason for such treatment is to prevent any loss of education from being unable to hear the teacher clearly. Evidence of any permanent damage to the ear from glue ear is patchy. Mind you, having your finger stuck in your ear for three weeks might be considered unusual behaviour so avoid superglue while fishing for wax.

Ear wax

All kinds of things can get into your ears. Earwigs are not
actually the most common visitor, although sleeping in a dahlia patch might be an offer they cannot
refuse. Fingers, cocktail sticks, cotton buds,
corkscrews, and match sticks are all regularly shoved
into people's ears to clean out wax. A patient once
came in and told me he could hear perfectly well
until he poked a length of fuse wire into his ear. 'I
was going crazy by the buzzing sound in my
ear after a day out in the country,' he said, 'so
I stuck a bit of 30 amp fuse wire in to see if it
made any difference.' It certainly did. I told him he had suc-
ceeded in impaling the beetle stuck in his ear wax but unfortunately he had also perforated his eardrum. Predictably he
replied, 'Pardon?' Not only had he damaged his eardrum,
the wire had also mangled up the tiny sensitive bones which
transmit sound vibrations to his brain.

Ear wax is produced in response to irritation. The more
you poke cotton buds in the ear, the more wax is produced.
This also goes for ear syringing. Never, ever let anyone
squirt water into your ear unless you know there is not a
hole in your eardrum. One of my patients with perforated
eardrums used to entertain his children by blowing bubbles
through his ears while lying
under water in the bath.
Unfortunately he had the
bright idea of sucking water
through his ears and
squirting it out again like
Moby Dick. Bath water,
especially his bath water,
is not the best thing with
which to rinse your ears out. All the ear wax in the world
could not prevent him from developing a nasty infection
which permanently damaged his hearing.

BOOM!

Cotton buds

Imagine an old cannon being loaded with a cannon ball. Trying to get ear wax out with a cotton bud is like trying to get a cannon ball out of a cannon with a ramrod. It simply pushes the wax even harder against the eardrum. Worse still, if water gets in there, it sits behind the wax and makes everyone sound as though they are talking through a blanket. Let your GP have a look. If it is really impacted, you can use softening eardrops which allows the wax to run out. Ear-syringing should never be done unless you can see the eardrum. Alternatively get your girlfriend to suck your ear. It will taste terrible but at least you will find out if she really loves you.

Incidentally, ear wax was used by Spanish conquistadors to stiffen their moustaches. History fails to relate just exactly whose ear wax was used and whether the ears were actually connected to their heads when the wax was removed.

Where did you get those peepers?

Now I don't want
you to tell
anyone else
about this, it's
rather
embarrassing.
A patient arrived
by ambulance to
casualty after a
road traffic accident. As she had
been knocked out, I used an
ophthalmoscope, a sort of small flat
telescope, to look at the back of her eyes.
Pressure building up inside the skull can
cause changes in the appearance of the
retina, which help to make a quick
diagnosis, which, in turn, can prevent
serious brain damage. As luck would have
it, I was also teaching medical students at

the time, so I laid on my most professional air. While I struggled to see into her left eye, she whispered in my ear, 'That's a glass eye, Doctor. I thought you might like to know.' Unfortunately she was also partly deaf, so her whisper could be heard as far as the waiting room.

The eyeball is roughly spherical, approximately 2.5 cm (1 in) in diameter, with a pronounced bulge of the cornea at the front. The innermost layer is the light-sensitive retina. The cornea is a tough, five-layered membrane through which light is admitted to the interior of the eye. Behind the cornea is a chamber filled with clear, watery fluid which separates the cornea from the lens. If the pressure in this fluid is not maintained at the right level, the retina can be destroyed, with complete loss of vision. Called glaucoma, this disease runs in families and you should have your eyes checked regularly if there is anyone in your family who suffered from it. The lens is connected by ligaments to a ring-like muscle which surrounds it. This muscle, by flattening the lens or making it more nearly spherical, changes the focus of the eye. The pigmented iris hangs behind the cornea in front of the lens and has a circular opening in its centre. The size of its opening, the pupil, is controlled by a muscle around its edge. This muscle contracts or relaxes, making the pupil larger or smaller, to control the amount of light admitted to the eye. When you find someone attractive it dilates, which explains why you always have such enormous pupils when you look in the mirror.

Behind the lens the main body of the eye is filled with a transparent, jellylike substance. The pressure of this goo keeps the eyeball distended. The retina is right at the back of the eye. It is a complex layer, composed largely of nerve cells. The light-sensitive receptor cells lie on the outer surface of the retina in front of a pigmented tissue layer. These cells take the form of rods or cones packed closely together like matches in a box. This layer can detach from its basal layer in some diseases or by trauma, producing a detached retina. Using laser, the retina can be 'welded' back on to the pigmented layer beneath. Where the optic nerve enters the eyeball, below and slightly to the inner side of the fovea, a small round area of the retina exists that has no light-sensitive cells. This optic disk forms the blind spot of the eye.

Focusing

A young child can see clearly at a distance as close as 6.3 cm (2.5 in), but with increasing age the lens gradually hardens, so that the limits of close seeing are approximately 15 cm (about 6 in) at the age of 30, and 40 cm (16 in) at the age of 50. In the later years of life most people lose the ability to accommodate their eyes to distances within reading or close working range. This condition, known as presbyopia, can be corrected by the use of special convex lenses for the near range. Structural differences in the size of the eye cause the defects of hypermetropia (farsightedness) and myopia (nearsightedness).

Protective structures

We have several structures to protect the eye. The most important of these are the eyelids. They protect against excessive light and trauma. The eyelashes, a fringe of short hairs growing on the edge of either eyelid, act as a screen to keep dust particles and insects out of the eyes when the eyelids are partly closed. As they are connected to the eyelid, they can be fluttered up and down, which may protect women from a parking ticket but can lead to severe nasal pain when performed by a man. The under surface of the eyelid is covered in a thin protective membrane, the conjunctiva, which doubles over to cover the visible part of the eye. Each eye also has a tear gland, or lacrimal organ, situated at the outside corner of the eye. The salty secretion of these glands lubricates the forward part of the eyeball when the eyelids are closed and flushes away any small dust particles or other foreign matter on the surface of the eye. The tears drain down into the nose, which is why your nose always runs when you reach the end of *Love Story*. Normally human eyelids close by reflex action about every six seconds, but if dust reaches the surface of the eye and is not washed away, the eyelids blink more often and more tears are produced. On the edges of the eyelids are a number of small glands, the Meibomian glands, which produce a fatty secretion that lubricates the eyelids themselves and the eyelashes. The eyebrows also have a protective function in soaking up or deflecting perspiration or rain and preventing the moisture from running into the eyes. They are also useful for expressing intense surprise, such as when you realise too late that there is no toilet paper left.

Eye diseases

Styes are common. They are an infection of the follicles of the eyelashes. Topical antibiotics and sometimes removing the eyelash which is in the centre of the stye can help. Entropion, the turning of the eyelid inwards toward the cornea, and ectropion, the turning of the eyelid outwards, can be caused by scars or from chronic irritation. The eyes tend to water and the tears spill down the face instead of into the nose. More seriously, the inward-turned eyelid can permanently scar the front of the eye affecting normal vision. Simple surgery will correct this. Conjunctivitis is simply any infection of the conjunctiva. It produces a crusty deposit which tends to glue the eyelids together after sleeping. Herpes is a virus which can infect the cornea and if not treated can permanently damage vision. If your eye is itchy, sore and red, see your doctor. Many people's eyes are occasionally red, more often on a Saturday morning. Macular degeneration, which affects the central retina, is the most frequent cause of loss of vision in some older people.

Contact lenses

The number of people wearing contact lenses instead of glasses has increased, so much so that an unconscious patient is always checked for lenses as they arrive in casualty. Soft lenses which absorb water are often more comfortable to wear but have a limited life as they tend to coat with protein which becomes increasingly difficult to remove. More importantly, they can lead to infection of the eye if not cared for properly – tap water is not a suitable storage medium and commercial preparations must be changed regularly. Oxygen permeable hard lenses allow the surface of the eye to 'breathe'. Don't forget, the reason why the front of the eye, the cornea, is transparent is because there are no blood vessels in it. It is supplied with oxygen and food through the tear fluid which covers the eye each time you blink. If you have difficulty in producing tears, as in Sjogren's syndrome, the eye can become opaque. One way of improving your flow of tears is to let your feet slip off the pedals while riding a bike with a crossbar. Never fails. That's why cyclists can see so well. Lenses you throw away each day are very safe, if a bit expensive.

Basically all lenses work the same way. Most problems with short sight are caused by an incorrect shape of the cornea. It is the difference in refraction between the air and the cornea which helps focus the image onto the retina at the back of the eye. This explains why you can only see properly if you wear goggles while swimming under water. By creating a tear film between the lens and the cornea, a contact lens changes the way the light is focused. If you perform tiny cuts on the surface of the cornea, the shape of the cornea changes as the cuts heal. The net result is like having contact lenses on all the time, but without the discomfort. By using laser, these fine cuts can be made very safely and can now be used to treat severe short sight.

Gnat a scratch – parasites

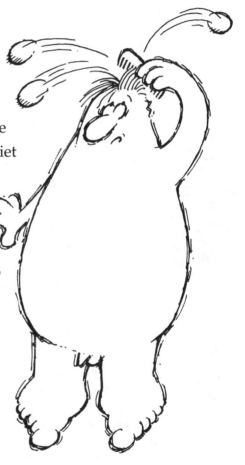

A patient once came in and shook my hand. As he held it he told me, in a quiet voice, that he had scabies. Indeed he did. Never in all my experience as a doctor have I ever seen so much scabie on so little human. This man had standing room only for scabies.

Parasites come in all shapes and sizes and have little regard for social class, religion or sex. Many a phone call has come from a posh person who would rather the receptionists didn't know they could feel the patter of tiny feet. The strangest thing is, I always get an itchy ear afterwards.

The largest parasites must be tapeworms. *Taenia soleum*, the pork variety, can grow almost as long as the gut itself. A knobbly head, or scolex, with hooked spines lodges itself into the gut wall of a human. The tapeworm then sheds its eggs into the faeces which end up on the grass *au naturel* and subsequently inside a pig. Once inside the stomach the eggs hatch and burrow to the brain, tongue or eyes. Eating these bits produces a form of pork scratchings you would rather do without. Luckily it is now very rare in the UK and even

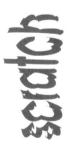

the more common beef tapeworm is easily treatable. Much more common is the threadworm, or roundworm, which is the length of your fingertip and thousands can live in the bowel. They are active at night, causing mind blowing itchiness at the anus. It tends to run in families and, except in badly debilitated people, they are harmless. One single dose of medicine (Vermox) is all that is required, although you can be reinfected after a week or so. It is recommended that all family members, whether obviously infected or not (except those who are under 2 years or pregnant), should be treated at the same time.

Smaller, and more mobile, are crabs and lice, which are essentially the same at a scratch. About the size of a large pinhead, they scuttle about in the hairy bits laying eggs on the hair shafts. It was the job of the 'nit-nurse' to metal-comb out these hangers-on after a good dose of DDT or Malathion had bumped off the parents. Unless they carry some disease from another person, they are relatively harmless.

Scabies is nasty. It is a skin disease caused by *Sarcoptes scaboi*, a mite smaller than a pinhead which burrows just under the skin causing an intense itch. If you look carefully you can see the little chap munching away in a long burrow.

In between your fingers and the back of your hands are its favourite pastures. Your doctor will prescribe a lotion and your clothes will need to be washed. Best to treat the whole family as it is extremely contagious.

The smallest parasites are bacteria and viruses. It makes sense for a parasite not to actually kill its host so eventually we tolerate each other. Scarlet fever used to be a major killer; Beth in *Little Women* died from it. Now it causes a minor rash. It just goes to show, parasites can grow on you.

I once knew a man who loved dogs so much he would kiss them right on the nose. On a holiday in France he did just that to a rather bedraggled-looking hound. It bit him right on the nose. Unfortunately the dog also had rabies and our dog lover had a nervous few weeks of injections and tests.

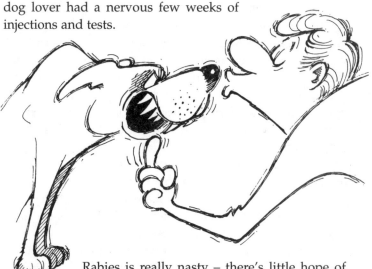

Rabies is really nasty – there's little hope of survival. The organism lives just as happily in dogs and foxes as it does in humans. Thankfully, most infections, however, are specific to particular species. The guy honking and snorting on the bus, for instance, is unlikely to have canine distemper. Unless, of course he happens to be a were-wolf.

Some bugs will live happily in more than one host. Rats can carry leptospirosis which causes the deadly Weil's disease. Stagnant water contaminated with rats' urine is the commonest source of infection. Colour-coded tops of milk once proudly proclaimed whether or not it was TT, tuberculin-tested. In fact most cases of tuberculosis are passed on from person to person.

One of the best-known bugs to travel well is salmonella. It is found living in a number of animals but where there is intensive farming it is difficult to eradicate. Chickens, and therefore eggs, can become infected and unless they are cooked thoroughly there is always the danger of food poisoning. You only find out that the egg or chicken you ate had a little lion inside it about two days after your meal. The vast majority of people survive, although babies, or chronically sick and debilitated people, are often not so fortunate.

Dog and cat fleas are a nuisance to people but can actually only survive with the pet around. Much more dangerous is the organism *Toxocara* which may be passed in their droppings. Cats find children's sandpits convenient. This particularly nasty bug causes blindness and is easily avoided by regularly worming your pets.

Sheep farmers occasionally pick up a viral infection called orf, especially on the back of their hands. It looks dreadful but in fact is relatively harmless and responds well to a treatment developed in London called 'Get orf'. Honest.

Those little worms you see on the gills of fish are harmless. Some of the bugs which live on the gills of shellfish, however, are not so benign. Rotaviruses can survive in brackish water. They are commonly found around the outlets of sewage drains. Shellfish filter out food from the surrounding sea using their gills. Unfortunately they also pick up the rotavirus, which doesn't give the cockle a profuse diarrhoea, just you.

In short, don't go around kissing noses, or gills for that matter.

The bald facts

I didn't recognise my patient when he first walked in. Instead of his usual Yul Brynner hairstyle, he looked as though a black cat had crawled onto his head and died of fright. The fact that his beard, which would have shamed Robinson Crusoe, was bright red did not appear to concern him. 'I am wearing a wig,' he told me, interrupting my call to the National Society for the Prevention of Cruelty to Animals. 'I am going for a new job and I thought I would look younger with a full head of hair.' It transpired that he wanted a hair restorer courtesy of the NHS.

Hair is funny stuff. It is essentially dead, except for the folli-cles. This is a happy coincidence, particularly for barbers who would otherwise need to use a general anaesthetic every time they gave a short back and sides. Strangely enough, women have as many hair follicles on their face as do men but as they lack testosterone it fails to grow in the same way. Hair usually contains pigment (except in the case of albinos) but sometimes also con-tains air bubbles that give it a sil-very colour. The shaft of the hair consists of modified skin cells arranged in columns surrounding a central core and covered with thin, flat scales. The root of each hair is con-tained in a tubular pit of the skin called the hair folli-cle. The hair grows from the bottom of the follicle; it is nour-ished by the blood vessels. A minute muscle, the arrector pili, is attached to each hair follicle to make the hair 'stand on end'. The rate of hair growth varies with the age of the person and with the length of the hair. When a hair is short, its rate of growth averages about 2 cm (about 1 in) per month; by the time the hair is 30 cm (12 in) long, the rate of growth is reduced by one half. The fastest growth is found in women from 16 to 24 years of age.

hair follicle

epidermis

dermis

arrector pi

blood vessels

Patterns of hair growth are complex and involve genetic traits. Men from some oriental parts of the world charac-teristically have little facial hair, while the Scandinavian males are epitomised by their great bushy beards. The form of the hair is one of the most important and reliable hereditary characteristics. The nearly black hair of the Papuan,

Melanesian and African grows from a curved follicle, which imparts a spiral twist, and is flat or tapelike in cross section. The hair of the Chinese, Japanese, and Native American is straight, coarse, and almost always black. It grows from a straight follicle and is round in cross section. The hair of the Ainu, European, Hindu, and Semite is wavy and intermediate between the straight and curly types. It grows from a straight follicle but has a slight tendency to curl; it is oval in cross section and among individuals exhibits a wide range of colour, from light blond to black.

Facial hair and scalp hair respond differently to testosterone. They even feel different. Scalp hair is softer and finer, while facial hair is coarser, like pubic hair. At the junction between the two types of hair, just in front of the ears, there is a sort of 'no man's land' where hair of either kind is often deficient. Fair hair makes this more obvious. Most men disguise this by growing their scalp hair slightly longer to cover this region of comparative baldness.

You might not think of being bald as a health risk, but one of my patients very nearly ceased to be simply out of the fear of going bald. He told me he was considering suicide because each time he checked in the mirror his hairline was receding like a spring tide. I have to say there were just about as many wrinkles on the beach too. Such concern is not uncommon. Biblical Elisha had a way with children who laughed at his bald head. He cursed them in the name of the Lord, whereupon, 'there came two she bears out of the wood and tore forty and two of them'. Try that on your kids next time they call you baldy bonce.

Men will go to extraordinary lengths and expense to prevent themselves shining. A top hair specialist in London had one man who asked for castration in order to save his hair. As luck has it, if anyone comes to me asking for the same, I still have two house bricks left behind by a vet but such treatment is very drastic and often unnecessary.

There are different types of baldness. Some are caused by ringworm infection and can be treated with a lotion from your GP. Alopecia areata is a baldness which can affect all the hair on the body, including the eyebrows. The cause is often never found and the hair often regrows. Nasty shocks are supposed to cause your hair to fall out. Luckily this is not true or every man with teenage children would look like Kojak after reading the telephone bill.

Chronic illness can affect hair growth, as can hormone changes. Chemotherapy can sometimes cause hair loss but radiotherapy only rarely does so. One old, and extremely dangerous, treatment for childhood scalp conditions was to irradiate the whole head, causing the hair to fall out and exposing the bare skin for treatment. Disorders of the hair shaft or hair follicle cause abnormal growth or premature falling of the hair. Certain conditions such as dull or dry hair are caused by physical or chemical agents. Too frequent use, for instance, of permanent-waving chemicals or of shampoos and lotions, especially those containing alcohol, often causes such conditions. The cause of excessive hairiness is obscure, but in several cases it has been traced to tumours of the adrenal cortex or to disorders of the pituitary gland, the thyroid gland, or the ovary. Premature greying of the hair is associated with anxiety, shock and deficiency diseases. Diffuse loss of the hair, ordinarily a normal phenomenon, may reach abnormal proportions after a fever higher than 39.4° C (103° F) or during a long debilitating disease. There is no evidence that you can lose all the hair on your head from a fright, unless of course you happen to be wearing a dead cat.

The commonest form of hair loss is male pattern balding. Testosterone is a factor. Hippocrates, the Greek doctor and philosopher, noticed that eunuchs not only had high voices, they also had a full head of hair. Just thinking about castration is enough to raise my voice a couple of octaves. As the testes produce testosterone, the explanation is obvious. Hair follicles, genetically programmed to be sensitive to testosterone, react to the hormone. Thus if your dad and his dad were bald in a particular way, then you can bet your hairy armpits you will be as well.

Treatment falls into three main camps. Transplant, drugs and disguise. Wigs can now be bought on hire purchase. So much down and so much toupee. Hair transplants are expensive but can be effective if you don't mind looking like Elton John. A more promising treatment involves *minoxidil*, a drug originally designed for high blood pressure. In some cases it can restore your lost hair but the treatment is life long. It is also expensive and cannot be obtained on the NHS. Sorry to be so blunt but these are the bald facts.

Liver, kidney and black pudding

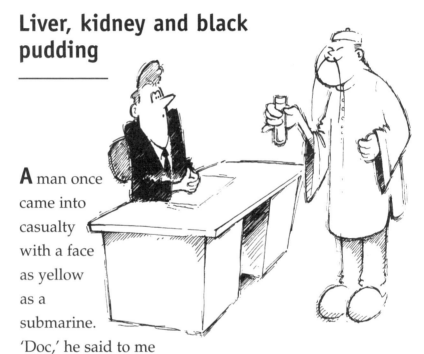

A man once
came into
casualty
with a face
as yellow
as a
submarine.
'Doc,' he said to me
in a thick, yellow accent, 'my wee has
turned yellow.' I believed him. Even his
eyes were yellow. You could have grated
him up and used him for saffron. He had
hepatitis, a liver condition.

Without the liver there would only be Pool FC and onions would never taste the same again. It sits just under the chest and contrary to what most men think it is the largest body organ. If you ever get the chance to be reincarnated as a bit of someone else, don't choose the liver. Bend an ear or pick a nose, anything but the liver. When it came to sorting out the jobs parts of the body have to perform, livers came off worst. Not only does it have to make proteins to keep the water in your blood and not in your socks, it also produces all the clotting agents. When a doctor asks, 'What's the bleeding time?' he is not looking forward to lying in a bed. Bleeding time is the time it takes for blood to clot. Liver damage prolongs clotting and with a complete lack of any one of the vital clotting factors, the blood just keeps flowing. Because of a genetic disorder, haemophiliacs lack the clotting agent Factor VIII. Affected people bleed into their joints with agonising results. It is possible to replace the missing factor from donated blood or increasingly from genetic engineering.

If you imagine a compost heap, you won't be a long way away from the liver. On go all the tea bags, grass cuttings, horse droppings and out comes lovely manure. The poor liver has to cope with all the toxins produced by the body, and get rid of the worn-out blood cells and turn them into something useful or at least less harmful. If it cannot

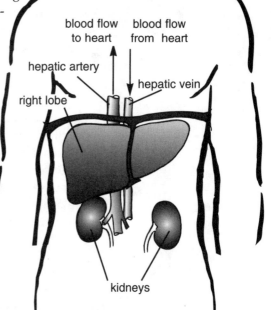

blood flow to heart   blood flow from heart

hepatic artery

hepatic vein

right lobe

kidneys

cope, yellow blood pigments build up in the skin and pass with the urine.

Alcohol is destroyed by the liver. Usually it does this with no problem. If too much too often comes along, however, damage occurs. 'Sod this for a lark,' it says. 'Get yourself a donor.' Fortunately the liver, unlike your brain, will regenerate if given the chance. A few days totally alcohol-free each week can do the trick.

Many drugs such as paracetamol are also destroyed by the liver but it only takes about 24 tablets within 12 hours to irreversibly wreck it. Death, never anything to write home about at the best of times, is particularly nasty after a paracetamol overdose. Young people will use paracetamol as a 'cry for help' not realising just how dangerous is this easily available medicine. Keep only small amounts and keep them safely locked away in the house.

Kidney donors

A patient once walked into casualty and asked to see the kidney-donor man. 'Look Doc,' he said in an agitated voice, 'I need a few bob, so I thought you might like one of my kidneys.' It's not every day you meet someone so generous.

Without kidneys we would all be eating steak and something else pie along with devilled nothings.

Almost the size of your fist, your kidneys lie just below the back of the ribcage. Never ask a boxer to show you where they are. They have a number of jobs, not least in excreting excess water, maintaining the correct balance of salts in the blood, stimulating the growth of blood cells and regulating blood pressure. All this and cheaper than a pound of steak. Marvellous. Most people have two, although you can wake up after a night out in some parts of the world with one missing. It wakes up in somebody else, usually a very rich somebody else. It is possible to have more than one duct, or ureter, draining each kidney to the bladder. Most people are never aware of this until something goes wrong. Renal colic is described as the 'worst pain known to man' but women suffer from it as well. Small stones form in the kidney and pass down the ureter. As it moves it scrapes the lining of the duct. Few painkillers will touch it. Most stones will make their own painful way out and rarely do any harm. In some cases it is necessary to remove the stone. A great deal depends upon where it is. By injecting a radio-opaque dye into the ureter, x-rays can show if a stone is causing a blockage. Under a general anaesthetic, a fine probe with a small basket is used to pull the stone down the ureter. Recently ultrasound has been used. Basically you sit in a bath and beams of ultrasound are focused on your stone which disintegrates. It's not painful but don't forget to wipe round the bath afterwards. If all else fails, surgeons will operate to remove the stone the hard way.

Kidney infections can be serious. Most people casually talk of having a chill on the kidneys but you certainly know about it when they are infected. Your temperature soars, blood is often passed as black clots in the urine and there is a constant dull low back pain. Antibiotics usually do the trick. If a ureter is blocked for a long time, or the urine passes backwards towards a kidney, it can cause hydronephrosis. The kidney gradually swells and becomes useless. Blood pressure can rise, causing damage to the remaining kidney. Unfortunately it is not always diagnosed until after the damage is done. Young children who develop a urine infection confirmed by analysis should therefore always be referred for investigation, to exclude such an abnormality.

Kidney donors save lives. Carry the card.

Blood brothers

I once knew a man who volunteered to donate blood. To give himself Dutch courage, he drank a bottle of whiskey, and fell over on his way to the transfusion centre cutting his wrists on a glass door. He needed three pints of blood when he came into casualty.

Blood really is a wonderful invention. It lets you know when the cheese has all been grated. If it were not for blood we would all look like Marcel Marceau. Red blood cells give the blood its characteristic colour. Called erythrocytes they are responsible for transporting oxygen around the body. Arterial blood rich in oxygen is bright red but turns a bluish tinge once it has dropped off its load. Carbon monoxide grabs hold of haemoglobin, a protein in the red blood cell which is responsible for oxygen transport. It never lets go. All the body can do is destroy the cell and use the bits to make a new one. Smoking produces gobfuls of this gas and thus limits efficient muscle action, particularly in the heart. Anaemia usually indicates a lack of red blood cells; on the other hand, it is possible to produce too many. This happens in heavy smokers or in a rare condition, haemochromatosis, which runs in families. A hormone, erythropoetin, is secreted by the kidneys, which stimulates the bone marrow to produce more red blood cells. This hormone can now be manufactured artificially. If your kidneys are removed for some reason, anaemia can be a complication, but treatable with erythropoetin.

White blood cells protect the body from infection. They are also produced in the bone marrow. The body codes these cells to recognise specific molecules called antigens found on the surface of bacteria and viruses. Should any of the white blood cells come into contact with these molecules, they trigger the production of more similarly encoded cells and the production of antibodies which enable the bacteria or viruses to be destroyed. Vaccination cons the body into thinking it has been invaded by a nasty. 'Ello,' says the white blood cell, 'I recognise this little bug 'ere' and promptly blows its bugle. Radiation, HIV and certain medicines used for treating cancer reduce the body's ability to fight disease. Bone marrow donors help restore the body's ability to produce white blood cells after such treatment. Contrary to popular belief, such donations are not agony and are incredibly simple. A large number of people owe their lives to such donors.

Small sticky cells called platelets help stop the loss of blood through a cut. They clump together blocking the hole. Too few of these cells, or a defect in the hormonal system which triggers clotting, can lead to bleeding inside the body.

Excuses for not donating blood are easy to find. Even though experiments with artificial blood are promising, the transfusion service still need thousands of pints every week. Blood donors save lives.

Getting under your skin

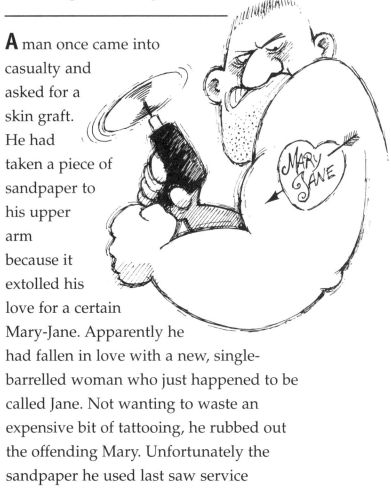

A man once came into casualty and asked for a skin graft. He had taken a piece of sandpaper to his upper arm because it extolled his love for a certain Mary-Jane. Apparently he had fallen in love with a new, single-barrelled woman who just happened to be called Jane. Not wanting to waste an expensive bit of tattooing, he rubbed out the offending Mary. Unfortunately the sandpaper he used last saw service

bringing up the best on an Austin Allegro
and he developed a nasty infection right
over the much lamented Mary. This has to
be the only sexually transmitted disease
ever caused by sandpaper.

Skin stops all your blood falling out – without it, we would
all look like raw hamburgers. It forms a protective barrier
against all the nasties, like bacteria. It also contains the special organs for the various sensations, such as sense of touch.
It is important in maintaining body temperature through
the activity of its sweat glands and blood vessels. One
square inch (6.5 sq. cm) of skin contains up to 15 ft (4.5 m) of
blood vessels, which get rid of excess heat by dilating.

Skin is composed of two distinct layers. The outer layer,
the epidermis or cuticle, is several cells thick and has an
external, horny layer of dead cells that is constantly shed
from the surface and replaced from below by a basal layer of
cells. If you close a room up completely it gathers no dust.
The reason is simple: most dust is, in fact, human skin. In an
experiment a woman volunteer used a vacuum cleaner on
her tights every day to see how much skin she lost.
In one month she filled a jam jar with dead skin.
Dust mites, you will be glad to hear, live on this
dead skin and their faeces causes asthma sufferers
and hypersensitive allergic people no end of misery.
You can buy special filters to go on your
vacuum cleaner to get rid of it out of
the carpet. Don't use a vacuum cleaner on your tights while you are wearing them. Neighbours talk, and
leaving the house with a vacuum
cleaner tube stuck up your trouser
leg can raise an eyebrow or two,
often on the same person.

The skin's inner layer, the dermis, is

composed of a network of collagen and elastic fibres, blood vessels, nerves, fat lobules, and the bases of hair follicles and sweat glands. Collagen provides elasticity and with age becomes stiffer, which makes skin floppy and loose. Vitamins A, E and C are said to help maintain skin turgidity. You will know if your skin is loose when you turn round too quickly and find yourself looking out of the back of your scalp.

dead cells

epidermis

dermis

sweat gland

hair follicle

blood vessels

fat lobules

Skin colour varies with the amount of pigment deposited in the skin cells. The colour also varies in some diseases or because of pigmented substances carried to it by the blood, as in jaundice. Mellow yellow can result from many diseases of the liver, which breaks down the blood pigments otherwise stored in the skin.

No sweat

With increased body temperatures there is an enhanced blood flow to the skin surface, which is why you go red when you are hot. When the temperature is low, blood vessels constrict to reduce blood flow and thus reduce heat loss. Temperature is regulated by a special centre in the brain. Glands in the skin secrete moisture, which, on evaporation, cools the body surface. We tend to forget that the skin is really a waste disposal machine and gets rid of many toxins by this route. Dogs can taste the difference between 'clean' sweat and sweat contaminated by toxins such as alcohol. Meat eaters actually smell different from vegetarians.

Sweat glands are found all over the body. There are more on the palms and soles but relatively few on the skin of the back. Sebaceous glands are sac-like glands that secrete the sebum that lubricates and softens the skin. They may also be responsible for secreting pheromones, otherwise known as sex attractants. Why on earth the largest number are found on the soles of the feet totally defeats me, if you will pardon the expression. Toe suckers rejoice. Incidentally did you know that the correct term for toe sucking is 'shrimping'? No, nor did I. Apparently it's due to the appearance of the little toe. Always cut your toenails before shrimping or you might just remove somebody's tonsils.

Skin diseases

Your skin is under attack from both inside and out. Dermatitis is just inflammation of the skin. It can result from exposure to irritating substances in industry or from contact with vegetable poisons, such as poison ivy. Skin infections are common but not usually serious. Impetigo, a crusty, scabby-looking infection, is often found in schools and also in rugby football players (scrumpox, in this case) and responds well to penicillin. Some illnesses of the body will show themselves on the skin. Measles, scarlet fever and chickenpox are all common. Telling the difference can be tricky but, generally speaking, measles starts behind the ears with distinct spots gradually merging, scarlet fever is a diffuse rash on the body, and chickenpox starts all over the body at the same time with intensely itchy pustules. Why the chicken crossed the road was probably to find a decent back-scratcher. Substances such as proteins, to which the body is unduly sensitive, may affect the skin by producing hives or weals. Fish, strawberries and bee stings can all affect the skin of sensitive people. We used to test for sensitivity in patients by placing a small amount of the suspect protein on a small scratch in the skin. Sensitivity was indicated by the appearance of a weal. This is less often routinely performed because of the danger of an overreaction which can even be fatal. Eczema, formerly considered the most common skin disease, is now regarded as a symptom of any of a variety of conditions, including external local irritations, disorders of the blood, and allergy.

Lumpy skin

Big lumps in the skin are common. The commonest cause are lipomas, globs of fatty tissue which can gradually increase in size from a pea to a tennis ball. Although totally harmless, they can be a nuisance. Your GP can remove them. Lumps on the neck, under the arms or at the groin deserve early attention from your doctor, as infection or cancer can enlarge the glands of the lymphatic system involved in protection from disease located in these areas.

More men than women suffer and die from cancer of the skin. There are now 50 new cases per 100,000 men each year in the UK. These are mainly squamous carcinomas, or basal cell carcinomas, which are eminently treatable. Melanoma, however, is also on the increase. It's not just sunny holidays to blame, either. Many men are at risk while living and working in the British Isles, not noted for a particularly sunny climate.

High risk

Some men are more at risk than others, especially those who have:

- A job which involves continuous exposure to sunlight, such as farmers, fishermen, builders or postmen.
- Had a previous cancer of the skin.
- A fair complexion or who burn easily in the sun. Black men are far less at risk than white men. Even so, it is still

possible to develop skin cancer, so you should protect your skin no matter what its colour.

- Numerous moles. Particularly so if they are already large, irregular in shape and have different colours. Even white moles can turn nasty, so keep an eye on them.
- A close relative, such as your father, brother, mother or sister, who has had skin cancer. There may be a link which runs in families.

Mole menace

Any mole which changes shape, colour or starts to bleed should be checked by your GP. Melanoma can make its presence known this way, and is very treatable when caught early. 'Skin aware' campaigns in Australia have helped save thousands of young males and females. Similarly, the persistent lump on the lower lip, forehead or tip of the ear which could be a squamous carcinoma or a basal cell carcinoma, should also be examined by a doctor. Treatment involves minor surgical removal of the lump and is invariably successful when caught early, so don't delay. Lumps have a nasty habit of growing on you.

Prevention

Skin cancer is neither inevitable nor rare. Prevention is not difficult:

- Always use a high factor sun block in strong sunlight. You don't have to be in sunny Spain to get an overdose of sun. Sunburn, which means you have badly damaged your skin, is common even on a holiday in the British Isles.
- Protect your head and face when working in the sun. Wear a hat with a wide brim – all the corks hanging down are optional extras.
- Be skin aware. Check your skin regularly, don't forget your back – get

someone to look for you or use a hand mirror.

- Watch moles carefully. If they change colour, increase in size, bleed, become painful, or if they change shape, consult your GP.

Sun learnt

For some men, being tanned is a big plus. 'To be honest, I actually liked coming home burnt after working in the sun. I felt healthier, as if I had got something for nothing,' said a young man in casualty. 'It was my girlfriend who noticed the mole on my back. It had become a big lump and was bleeding every time I took my shirt off.' He had developed a melanoma from frequent exposure to the sun. Luckily it was caught in time and he survived. Protecting your skin makes sense.

Pure graft

Burns can wreck large areas of skin and the only way of repairing it is to skin-graft. Sections of skin of either full thickness or partial thickness are cut from another part of the body (the donor site) and applied to the raw surface (the recipient site), to which they usually stick. Eventually the graft merges with the surrounding skin to cover the entire area.

Only your own skin will do, although if you are an identical twin you might be able to entice them into the shower and give them a good rubbing over with a Ladyshave. Your body's immune system won't ever know the difference. Your brother, on the other hand, might just get an inkling that all is not as it should be and never watch *Psycho* ever again.

The unkindest cut of all

A young man once came into casualty with a nasty cut to his face. 'Don't worry,' says I, 'using a special method of stitching, you won't even see the scar.' He looked as though his granny had just died. 'But Doc,' he complained bitterly, 'can't you make it really gruesome looking?' I successfully resisted the temptation to sew his top lip to his eyelid.

Cuts can be dangerous. Soil and cars are covered in tetanus bugs. Keep your shots up to date, particularly if you are a farmer or a mechanic. Lock jaw gets its name from the tetanic muscle spasm which gradually works its way up to the brain. By the time your jaw muscles have locked, it is getting a little late to order a last meal.

Infection can set in if a wound is not cleaned properly. You don't need to use antiseptics, bleach or even a single malt whisky. Tap water will do well and it doesn't kill all the good-guy bugs which live on the skin and actually prevent infection from the bad guys. If you are caught a long way from a hospital with a nasty wound, pour a big dollop of sugar into it. This bumps off bacteria a treat but tends to flavour your tea if you reuse it. The ancient Greeks used honey for the same reason. Ironically, wounded soldiers left on the battlefield for a few days often survived better than those taken immediately to field hospitals. Maggots ate away the dead meat, preventing gangrene. This is now the basis of a modern treatment for leg ulcers. You can get lovely juicy maggots from your local angler's supply shop. Next time you cut yourself shaving forget about little pieces of toilet paper, slap on a handful of maggots. Don't forget to kiss your wife as you leave for work.

Closing the wound is important. It prevents infection and stops any further bleeding. If the cut is in the scalp it can produce an impressive amount of blood. We once used silk stitches to close the wound. Now you are more likely to come out of casualty with a row of stainless steel staples in your head. Superglue is often used on children which is painless and quick. Care is needed applying the glue to the hair. I once had to have a small child cut off my fingers.

Falling on to a dirty road can not only cut the skin, it can

Do not try this at home!

also impregnate the skin with gravel and muck. Unless this is cleaned out properly, it will cause a permanent 'tattoo'. Dog bites and especially human bites cannot be stitched completely because teeth are covered in harmful bugs, and tight-stitching the wound only traps the bugs under the skin, causing a deep-seated infection. Always carry a toothbrush in case a Rottweiler is about to bite your leg off. We can sew your hand back on at the same time.

Warts can grow on you

I used to know a man who could charm warts off anybody. You paid him a shilling and he charmed your warts off you for sixpence apiece. Apparently it worked, because I have never seen a human being so badly covered in warts. On the day he died all his old clients suddenly developed a wart on their nose . . .

The common wart is caused by the papilloma virus. It claims squatters' rights by invading skin cells and convincing them to time-share. 'Hey man,' says the wart, 'get a life. Get real. Be a wart.' This is an offer few skin cells can refuse and a proliferation of time-share, warty volcanoes is the result. Some con trick.

Warts are infectious, but not nearly as much as once thought to be. They are not a sign of poor personal hygiene and are extremely common. You can grow them anywhere there is skin. Verrucas are just warts forced to grow inwards.

Treatment has not changed much. You can have them removed with liquid nitrogen or burnt off with what is essentially an expensive soldering iron. Most lotions contain salicylic acid which attacks any skin, so you need to protect normal skin from the treatment. A corn plaster is a good way of keeping the lotion only on the wart. Silver nitrate sticks burn away the wart and can be very effective, but they can also damage the surrounding skin if not used properly. It is possible to develop warts on the skin of the penis. These are best removed by your doctor or at a genito-urinary clinic.

There is good evidence that warts have a cycle and will eventually disappear on their own. However, I find they need a bit of encouragement to vacate the premises. Your GP can help, and it is a good idea to get rid of small warts early on before they become unsightly. Children can be merciless in taunting other children with warts. Incidentally, swinging a dead cat around your head in a graveyard at midnight doesn't work. It also got me into terrible trouble with the NSPCA.

Dangerous liaisons –
STDS

A man once came into casualty and complained of catching vernacular disease off his girlfriend. Funny enough, he swore blind that he hadn't slept with anyone else, so I suppose he must have been right. Terminology moves on, often leaving confusion in its wake. Diseases you caught during sex used to be called venereal diseases or VD. This actually only referred to syphilis and gonorrhoea. Progress in the area now means you can catch much more than just these two, so the term has been replaced by 'sexually transmitted diseases' which covers everything. The abbreviation STD has stuck and is now the accepted term.

As usual, men come top of the class for catching STDs. Worse still, four times more men are contracting sexually transmitted diseases than were in 1975. A rough estimate puts the figure each year in the UK at around 35,000 men. This figure is based on attendance at genito-urinary clinics in England and Scotland and does not include those men who only attended their GPs. The true figure may be even greater because some men do not realise they are infected as they have no symptoms. Luckily not all the infections are dangerous, but some will most definitely kill. Despite all the advertising, the use of condoms, which gives almost 100 per cent safety from the real killers, is still not widespread enough to prevent the figures rising even further.

Misconceptions

Nothing is guaranteed to cause more mistrust and friction in a steady relationship than the sudden appearance of an STD. It can be difficult to convince your partner that you do not have to be unfaithful to get a dose. Thrush is a good example. It can be considered a sexually transmitted disease, as you can be infected during sexual intercourse. It also, however, can appear spontaneously often after prolonged use of antibiotics. Both partners need to be treated to eradicate the infection. Many other STDs can lie dormant and reappear years after they first developed.

In confidence

Some diseases are more socially acceptable than others. STDs come into the latter category for most people. The irony is that STDs are so common – most men who have been active sexually will have had a form of sexually transmitted bug at some time without realising it. Despite its prevalence, as with any other disease, people demand absolute confidentiality, and rightly so. Your GP fully understands this but if you want to be totally sure you can attend your local genito-urinary clinic and use a false name or a number or even no identification at all. This is considered quite acceptable. The staff are not allowed to tell even your own GP that you attended, or insurance companies, or employers or the police *even if you are under the age of consent*. The clinic will ask you to take part in confidential partner notification to help stop the spread of the particular STD from which you are suffering. Of one thing you can be assured: no one in a genito-urinary clinic is going to judge you, laugh at you or make you feel 'dirty'. These nurses and doctors are specially trained in the area but much more importantly, they are empathic and understanding. You will be treated as if you had just broken your finger, less painful too.

HIV and AIDS

Never has a single disease captured the imagination and exposed the thinly disguised prejudice endemic in our society as has Acquired Immune Deficiency Syndrome – AIDS. Following infection with the Human Immunodeficiency Virus (HIV), the white blood cells CD4 are depleted thus lowering the body's resistance to infection. At least 13 million people in the world today are HIV positive. Although the virus only appeared in the British Isles in 1982, there are over 4,000 new cases reported each year in the UK, with perhaps ten times this number undetected and undiagnosed. By 1997 the British Department of Health predicts that HIV-related death will be the third greatest cause of death in people under the age of 65 years. Despite controversy following reports in the popular press, designed more to sell newspapers than present the facts, HIV is not confined to gay men. It is on the increase amongst heterosexual men and intravenous drug abusers.

Symptoms like the tip of an iceberg

The early stages of infection generally go unnoticed and an antibody test from a blood or saliva sample is needed to confirm the presence of the virus. The appearance of the antibodies can take months and is known as seroconversion. A vague, non-specific illness similar to flu or glandular fever sometimes follows the initial infection after an interval of around six to seven weeks. A considerable period of time, years even, can then pass completely symptom free. The occurrence of oral thrush, persistent herpes (cold sores), or strange chest infections which only clear slowly with treatment are ominous signs of the body's declining ability to fight off other infections.

How to get it

Body fluids are often cited as the carrier of the virus. Actually this can be narrowed down to blood, semen and saliva. Although infection from saliva is extremely small, it makes sense to avoid obvious risks such as oral sex without adequate protection. There are no cases of doctors passing on the virus to their patients; although, conversely, a number of doctors have been infected by their patients. The main routes of infection are:

- Sexual transmission via blood from small cuts either in the mouth (oral sex), vagina, anus or penis. Sexual orientation is not exclusive, with both gay and straight men at risk.

- Blood transfusion in countries with poor medical resources is still a risk and you can buy a travel kit from your GP.
- Sharing dirty needles, razor blades, or even toothbrushes when there is bleeding from the gums.

According to the World Health Organisation up to 90 per cent of those people infected in the world contracted HIV through heterosexual sex of whatever form. Dental dams, 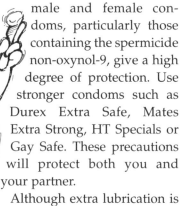 male and female condoms, particularly those containing the spermicide non-oxynol-9, give a high degree of protection. Use stronger condoms such as Durex Extra Safe, Mates Extra Strong, HT Specials or Gay Safe. These precautions will protect both you and your partner.

Although extra lubrication is often required during sexual activity, do not use an oil based lubricant such as Vaseline, baby oil, margarine or butter. They will damage the condom. There are water-based lubricants available such as KY Jelly or Foreplay. If you are not sure, ask the chemist; they sell thousands of these products and will not be embarrassed to give advice.

For more information, see the section 'Living with HIV' on page 172.

Other sexually transmitted diseases

Hepatitis B

One of the more deadly sexually transmitted diseases, hepatitis B, now has a protective vaccine. The number of infected men, however, is rising steadily in the UK and stands at roughly 700 men each year. Its effect can range from a flulike illness to total destruction of the liver. Typically it will cause varying degrees of jaundice – the yellowing of the skin and the whites of the eyes. This is caused by a build up of a pigment which is normally broken down by the liver.

Most men will not require immunisation but, depending on your life style, it may be wise to consult your GP. Hepatitis B is transmitted in the same way as HIV; that is, via the body fluids. There is evidence which suggests it is easier to become infected by the hepatitis B virus than by the virus that causes AIDS. Indeed, it only requires a tiny fraction of a drop of blood to transmit hepatitis B. For this reason, when there is bleeding from the gums, it can be caught from sharing a toothbrush or kissing. Worse still, the virus can survive a week or more in the dried state, so it can be picked up from a razor, for instance. Like HIV infections, there is no way of knowing if your sexual partner is infected with the hepatitis B virus. The incubation period (the length of time it takes before the illness manifests itself) is six months from infection. Some people can 'carry' the virus and yet not exhibit the condition. You cannot tell if a person is a carrier simply from their appearance; a blood test is required to be certain.

Genital herpes

This is the third most common STD, affecting roughly 11,000 men each year in the UK. It is on the slow increase with around 12,000 men infected in 1994. Doom and gloom once pervaded the scene when herpes was discussed. In fact, roughly 50 per cent of people who have had one attack never have another. Nevertheless, it is impossible to get rid of the virus completely. Herpes Simplex Virus (HSV) comes in two forms, HSV I and HSV II. Both will infect the same places and have a predilection for parts of the body where two types of skin meet together. The corners of the mouth, the outer parts of the genital areas and even the anus can be infected by both forms, although the type II herpes can be more dangerous, as it can affect the brain, causing a form of meningitis. Fortunately this is a rare complication.

Both types cause crusted blisters and then ulcers which

weep a thin watery material. This is highly infectious as it contains the virus which causes the condition. Coming in attacks which can last for months and then disappear for years or never return, you are definitely infectious during the presence of the sores. For some men the condition will pass unnoticed with only tiny ulcers on the penis to show its presence. Even when sores are not present, it might be possible to pass on the infection. Stress and coincidental illness can bring on these attacks.

Treatment

Acyclovir is a drug which can be applied directly to the affected skin or taken orally. It is most effective when the sores have yet to break out which is heralded by a tingling, itchy painful sensation in the affected area. While controlling the condition, acyclovir will not provide a cure and will be needed once again for any subsequent attacks. You need to arrange your sex life around the condition if you are having symptoms, as these mean you are highly infective. Condoms with a spermicide appear to offer greater protection against herpes infection than those without.

Genital warts

Papilloma viruses which cause warts will affect any part of the skin. The virus can be transmitted by physical contact, including sexual intercourse. Like warts commonly seen on hands, when on the penis they can vary in size from tiny skin tags to large fungating masses reminiscent of cauliflowers. While the latter are hard to miss, the less obvious form can be prevented from causing infection only by covering the affected area completely. One in eight people attending genito-urinary clinics will have genital warts. Around 50,000 men are treated for these warts each year in the UK, many more may simply put up with them. They usually cause little discomfort, although they are often itchy and may bleed with scratching. It is still not certain if they are a factor in causing cervical cancer in women and rectal cancer in women and gay men.

Treatment

There are drugs which can be applied directly to warts which will cause them to disappear. Liquid nitrogen is now used less often, as it can leave a painful 'burn' in such sensitive areas. Use a condom to prevent catching them in the first place.

Syphilis

As the English used to refer to this disease as the 'French pox', it seems only reasonable that the French referred to it as the 'English pox'. It takes, as they say, two to tango. Although a potentially serious condition, syphilis is now rare in the UK, with around 900 men infected each year. It is caused by a spirochaete, a microscopic parasite, which is highly infectious. Most men are unaware of being infected and complain of a painless ulcer on the penis around two weeks after intercourse. Detection becomes even more difficult when the ulcer disappears; the only sign of infection can be a fine rash over the body. If not treated, this can develop over a number of years into a condition which can affect the brain. Women show few signs of the infection in the early stages, except for small ulcers around the vagina, so it can easily go unnoticed by her sexual partner. The parasite cannot pass through a condom which will give almost 100 per cent protection.

Treatment

There are numerous horror stories about men having penicillin injected directly into their penises. In fact, the penicillin which is given as a single large dose can be given by injection to any part of the body and will invariably cure the condition if caught in the early stages.

Chlamydia

Non-specific urethritis, which simply means an inflammation or infection of the urethra (urinary passage in men), is an all-embracing term which includes infection by chlamydia. Men suffering from this infection complain of an intense burning sensation when passing water. There may also be a white discharge from the penis. It actually causes few problems for men other than this discomfort but can be disastrous if it is passed on to women. Not only is it the single biggest cause of infection of the fallopian tubes (pelvic inflammatory disease) leading to infertility and ectopic pregnancy (a potentially lethal condition where the egg attaches to the wall of the fallopian tube instead of the wall of the womb) but it can cause blindness and pneumonia in the child born to an infected woman. Thankfully rare in the British Isles, this is one of the major causes of childhood blindness in the world.

Condoms provide almost perfect protection.

Treatment

Symptoms of severe burning on passing water should be investigated by your doctor as it is eminently treatable with antibiotics.

Trichomoniasis

Causing a yellow-green discharge from the penis, this microscopic parasite lives in the urinary tract and usually causes pain during urination. On the other hand, it can be completely symptomless. When it has no effect on the male partner, but the female partner complains of a smelly green discharge from the vagina, tests may show its presence in the man.

Treatment

The parasite is sensitive to the antibiotic metronidazole (Flagyl) which is widely used. As it is related to a drug once used to treat alcoholics by making them violently sick should they revert to drinking, it is no surprise that the same can occur with metronidazole. Alcohol should be avoided with any antibiotic and can actually be dangerous with Flagyl.

Gonorrhoea

Caused by a bacterium, gonorrhoea is commonly misdiagnosed as often only minimum symptoms are apparent. It is commonly known as 'the clap', from the Old French *clapoir* meaning 'venereal sore'. This disease is not rare, as the 7,500 men who are infected each year in the UK will testify. It can cause a yellow-white discharge from the penis along with pain on passing water. When the anus is infected there can be a similar discharge. Most of the initial symptoms will start within five days of infection and include a vague polymyalgia, an ache of the joints and muscles. Although these symptoms can disappear after a further ten days or so, the man remains infectious. Gonorrhoea can cause reduced fertility in women if not treated.

Treatment

Antibiotics are usually effective. Condoms provide almost 100 per cent protection from infection.

Thrush

Contrary to popular belief, this common condition also infects men. Caused by a yeast, *Candida albicans*, thrush has the honorary title of being a sexually transmitted disease and is common among couples where there is no other sexual partner involved. Frequently the female partner will develop the symptoms, and will be treated by her doctor only to find them back again. Unlike the creamy discharge and intense irritation women usually experience, men may often have no idea that they are infected. Thus the infection continues to be passed on to the woman after each successive treatment. When it does make its presence felt in men, thrush causes a white discharge under the foreskin and a mild irritation over the head of the penis which may be worse during urination. Occasionally the head of the penis can appear mottled with a red blotch.

Treatment

Thrush responds well to antifungals which can be applied topically or taken orally. It is prone to reappear, particularly if you are taking numerous courses of antibiotics which tend to upset the natural balance of the body's commensal organisms.

scratch scratch scratch

Pubic lice

As you read this section you will begin to scratch. Each year 5,000 men in the UK will be scratching for the right reason. These tiny crablike, yellow-grey parasites attach themselves to the pubic hairs and live on blood sucked from the skin cut by their claws. It is for this reason that they are intensely itchy.

They only live for about 10 days but before the female dies she will lay around 3 to 4 eggs (nits) on the pubic hairs which then go on to increase the population. They are closely related to the louse, which infests the hair of the face and head, and can be treated in exactly the same way. Close body contact, such as intercourse, will provide the bridge for them to cross, but soiled sheets or towels will also transport them to your body. Although the merest thought of them provokes shudders in most people, they are actually relatively harmless except when they provide a route for the infection of more serious organisms, such as bacteria that cause abscesses.

SEAFOOD DRESS...

Treatment

Both partners, and the immediate family, should be treated with a special lotion or shampoo. You do not have to shave your pubic hair. Check with your GP which lotion to use. All bedding and clothes should be carefully washed and if necessary the mattresses should also be treated, as it requires only a small number to survive to cause reinfestation.

Keeping it up

A man once came into my surgery and told me he was having trouble getting it up. He was only mildly surprised by my usual let's-have-a-look-in-your-boxers approach, considering he was referring to a painful wrist and its effect on his golf.

Society places a certain importance to the size of a man's penis. While there is great variation in size throughout the animal kingdom, humans come top of the list in their group, the primates.

The penis also appears to have a disproportionate influence over the everyday life of the species, as few other animals give sex, as distinct from reproduction, the same level of priority; its role is complex and extends beyond the simple means of transferring sperm to the female or of passing urine. The Central Intelligence Agency, for example, seriously considered supplying oversized condoms to villagers during the Vietnam/Cambodian war to enhance the 'prowess' of American troops in the eyes of the enemy.

Average sizes

While men are prone to exaggerate, the average size of the human penis is actually around 7.5 cm (3 in) to 15 cm (6 in). There are operations which can lengthen the penis by up to 50 per cent, as almost half the penile structure is hidden within the pelvis. By cutting the ligaments which tether the penis to the pubic bones, the true length can be exposed. The only serious side effect of this procedure is the alteration in the angle of dangle. Instead of the erect penis standing to attention, it tends to take a more horizontal position. This is not said to adversely affect sexual pleasure. Numerous studies, however, have shown that penile length is not the main factor for sexual pleasure in the female or the male partner.

Boneless

Unlike some mammals, there is no bone in the human penis. Its function depends upon hydraulic pressure. Just as a balloon filled with water is more rigid than one without, the erect penis uses the same principle, using blood rather than water as the stiffening medium. By allowing blood into spongy tissue within the penis, but restricting its exit, the penis can enlarge by around 5 cm (2 in) during an erection. While valuable for placing sperm well into the vagina, an erection hinders the passing of urine. Indeed, there is a one-way valve at the base of the penis which prevents urine being passed at the same time as sperm. Urine or sperm travel down the penis from the bladder or from the testes in a narrow tube called the urethra. The thin skin of the penis is covered in small bumps which may be important in stimulation of the sexual partner. They also cause an unnecessary amount of concern, particularly amongst young men. These are the sweat glands and hair follicles that are not normally felt on thicker skin. They are even more noticeable during an erection because the skin is stretched even thinner.

bladder

prostate gland

urethra

penis

testicles (testes)

scrotum

Impotence

Penile erectile dysfunction is not the same thing as infertility. A man can father children without being able to have an erection. Problems with erections are common. A study in 1994 showed that in Britain at least 1 man in 4 has had some sort of erectile dysfunction at some stage in their lives. Furthermore, around 1 man in 20 has permanent erectile dysfunction problems. Misery on this scale is often masked by men's understandable reluctance to discuss these problems, despite the fact that many of them can be overcome by relatively simple treatments. For most cases of erectile dysfunction there will be a varying mixture of physiological and psychological causes, along with causes due to adverse affects of medicines. Around one third to one half of all cases will be purely psychological and will often respond well to non-clinical treatments such as sex counselling. Even though you may be unable to have an erection during attempted intercourse, if you have erections at any other time, then you have a psychological rather than physiological problem. For instance, you may be having erections in the middle of the night when you are asleep – this can be confirmed by your partner. Although there are scientifically based measuring techniques available to check nocturnal happenings you can always resort to the age-old method first devised at the time of the Penny Black. Stick a row of postage stamps around the shaft of your penis before retiring for the night while wearing a pair of underpants. If you have an erection the stamps will tear at the perforations making them still usable the following day. Just in case it doesn't work it might be advisable to use second class stamps. Successful erections during television programmes, sexy videos or masturbation bode well for the future, although it is not a 100 per cent test. You can either ask your GP for advice or contact the addresses listed on pages 196–9.

Psychological v. physiological causes

Counsellors can help with the problem of impotency. You will need to be honest with yourself and your counsellor, who will want to know a number of important things.

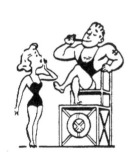

- Your life style: particularly, how much stress are you coping with? Do you consume much alcohol? Have you suffered a bereavement recently?
- Your childhood experiences and your attitude to sexuality. This may well include the attitudes of your partner.
- Your sexual experience during adolescence.
- Your own body image and how you feel about your genitals.
- How content you are with your sexual relationships.
- Bad trips. Have you had some painful experiences which are flavouring your appreciation of sex?
- Your feelings about sexual arousal. What is 'normal' or 'acceptable' practice for you?
- How you rate yourself as a sexual being.

After looking into these areas your counsellor will want to know if your present problems came on suddenly, and what preceded them. Psychological problems tend to come on quite abruptly, whereas physiological causes tend to be more insidious. Your medical history will be examined. Some medicines can cause erectile problems. Even homeopathic treatments can be a factor. Some diseases that travel in families, such as diabetes, hypertension or depression, can also be an important clue to diagnosis. Obviously details of drinking habits (remember brewer's droop?) and even smoking, diet and exercise can all be important.

Examination

A number of tests can be performed to exclude physiological causes. These include tests for:

- Diabetes.
- Anaemia.
- Liver problems.
- Thyroid deficiency. The thyroid is a gland in the neck that acts as a thermostat for body metabolism. If it is set 'too low' then everything slows down, including erections.
- Testosterone, prolactin and luteinising hormone levels. The balance between all three show if you are producing the right levels of hormone to make erections possible in the first place.

Your doctor will also check on your blood circulation. Poor blood flow through arteries in your legs can also mean the same thing for your penis. Your legs use bone to stay straight, your penis can only use the pressure of blood. He will also check on loss of facial hair, large breasts or small testes. These all indicate a hormone problem.

Age: the great escape

If ever there was a universal scapegoat for things that go wrong with the human body, particularly sexual activity, it has to be 'too many birthdays'. At last we are realising that sex is not just for the young and the enjoyment of sex can go on indefinitely.

Age-related problems associated with impotency do exist, but they are by no means its major cause. However, some important facts have emerged with recent studies. As we get older:

- There is a gradual decline in testosterone levels and the effect this hormone can have on target organs such as the penis.
- Erections take longer to develop and may require more tactile stimulation. Yes, the old Bentley may take longer to start than the new Porsche but it will give you a more comfortable ride. Might not run out of petrol so soon either.
- Self-image and concerns over sexual activity tend to be problems in later life. Men are notoriously bad at confronting these problems and will often let age take the blame.
- Physical illnesses take their toll on sexual activity, not least by the drugs which are commonly prescribed by way of treatment. We do tend to accumulate chronic conditions as we age.
- Prolonged periods without sexual activity can take their toll on sexual confidence. These periods may be due to bereavement, illness of a partner or divorce, and so on.
- Men are slow to admit depression to their doctors; older men even more so. Depression is a major factor for erectile dysfunction.

Common medicines and alcohol can be a factor

Some medicines are known to cause problems with erections:

- Some antidepressants are capable of making erectile dysfunction even worse. Talk to your doctor.
- Some antihypertension drugs for high blood pressure are common culprits. ACE inhibitors, alpha- and beta-blockers, and calcium channel blockers can all cause problems for certain individuals. You can change your medicine to help. See your GP.
- Alcohol is a common cause. Obviously binge-drinking has an immediate effect but chronic alcohol abuse can lead to permanent problems with erectile dysfunction. Small amounts of alcohol in the blood (up to 25 mg per 100 ml, one pint or one short, say) make erections easier. Levels greater than this cause the dreaded droop.

Common disease culprits

Diseases which affect the nerves or the blood supply can also cause problems. Multiple sclerosis is the most common spinal cord disease causing erectile dysfunction. There can also be bladder problems. Diabetes can cause a peripheral nerve problem which affects the ability to have an erection. Injections of a drug called papaverine straight into the spongy tissue of the penis can mimic the way the nerves work by restricting the blood flow out of the penis, thus producing an erection in men with this type of problem. It is surprisingly free of pain, although most men cross their legs just thinking about it.

Vascular problems account for around 25 per cent of erectile dysfunction in men. It usually has an insidious onset and is made worse by the consumption of even small amounts of alcohol. Injections of papaverine will not help as there is insufficient blood pressure to maintain an erection. Surgical implants are a possible answer.

Cancer of the penis

Penile cancer is thankfully rare. One or two men per 100,000 will develop the cancer and approximately 100 men will die each year in the UK. It is a disease of older men, usually over 65 years of age. If caught early it is eminently treatable with a 90 per cent survival rate. Despite this, many men consult their doctors too late.

Causes

Smegma, the cheesy secretion found under the foreskin, may be a culprit. Circumcised men rarely develop the tumour and it is almost unheard of in men circumcised at birth. It follows that personal hygiene is considered important.

Check it out

Carefully check the region between the glans (the head of the penis) and the foreskin. Look for small, often painless, ulcers or warty nodules. Difficulty in retracting the foreskin may indicate tethering at this point. A persistent red velvet-like patch on the glans needs medical attention even if it is painless.

Safe but scary

Tiny bumps all over the shaft are just sweat glands. Bleeding from beneath the foreskin after vigorous sex or masturbation is common – the skin between the foreskin and the glans is easily torn. If it persists see your doctor. It is easy to bruise the skin in the same way, with dramatic purple patches appearing the next day. They should disappear in a few days.

Treatment

Anti-cancer drugs can be applied as a paste to the tumour

Check it out!

itself. Localised radiotherapy and laser surgery are also used. Advanced cases require partial amputation, a couple of centimetres back from the growth. Cosmetic surgery restores normal services in the sex and waterworks departments. More advanced cases involve total amputation and the days of hitting flies on the wall are gone for ever.

Keep an eye on what is under the fly on your trousers, or buy a swatter.

When all else fails

Even when sex therapy, counselling, injections, three of sand and one of cement have failed, there is still a way of artificially producing a stiff penis for intercourse. Some will laugh at these treatments but they should remember how important sex is, not only to the average man but also to their partners. Relationships can be under immense strain and men even commit suicide over the inability to perform sex.

Vacuum devices

Vacuum devices have been around for over seventy years. They work by drawing blood into the penis under a gentle vacuum produced by a sheath placed over the penis and evacuated with a small pump. By restricting the blood's exit with a tight rubber band at the base of the penis, a respectable erection can be produced. It makes sense to remove the band after 30 minutes or so to avoid problems with blood clotting. These devices can be used by men with vascular problems. Your GP will be able to advise you on suppliers.

Penile implants

If there is no response to injections, a penile prosthesis may be the answer. Before you go down this road both you and your partner need to fully understand what is involved. There is a certain sacrifice of dignity which both of you will need to come to terms with. Having said that, many couples find the release of sexual frustration far outweighs the temporary embarrassment. There are three versions of implantable devices:

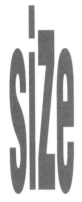

- Semi-rigid rods, made of silicone and sometimes covered with stainless steel braiding, are inserted into the spongy tissue of the penis.
- Two-cylinder, self-contained pumps are inserted into the penis and filled by squeezing the reservoir in the base of the penis.
- Inflatable penis prostheses consist of a pair of inflatable silicone cylinders implanted in the penis which can be filled by squeezing a pump implanted in the scrotum.

They all work, but as the old saying goes, 'It's not the size, it's what you do with it that counts.' Foreplay, sexual experimentation, avoidance of routine and being honest with each other is just as important as having a usable erection. Oh yes, and a healthy dollop of a sense of humour too. Sex, after all, is not only enjoyable it can be good fun as well. Noisy too.

Aphrodisia

Three thousand years ago the Chinese Emperor Chou Hsin was faced with impotence. Bad news for anyone, but this guy would balance a naked woman on his erect penis for the entertainment of his court. To restore his prowess he resorted to an aphrodisiac containing rhino tusk, and this substance is still considered by some to be potent medicine. Worse news for the rhino which now faces extinction. In her book, *A to Z of Aphrodisia*, (Thorsons) Diana Warburton reckons that even nettles can reach those places lagers also reach. Seventeenth-century gallants were advised to put a bunch of nettles in their codpiece, 'for the erection of the yeard to synne'. All this at a time when man-sized paper tissues hadn't even been invented.

If you don't happen to have a codpiece, stew a handful of carefully washed nettles in milk. Alternatively glaze a chopped onion in butter. Add three large handfuls of nettles. Steam for three minutes. Add a pint of milk, nearly boil, then liquidise. Cooking destroys the sting. Tastes delicious.

Spanish fly is well known and acts by irritating the mucous membrane lining the urethra in the penis. It is derived from crushed cantharis beetles. Unfortunately the itch persists after orgasm, often driving the user to distraction. Men have died from this stuff, but usually with a smile on their face.

According to Warburton, oysters resemble female genitalia. Greeks and Romans knew their value and enormous quantities were transported from Colchester to Rome. The Emperor Vitellius ate up to 1,000 at each sitting. *Up Pompeii* might not be too far from the truth after all. For the sake of science I once ate 23 live oysters. I counted them going in and I counted them coming back and it was the same number.

Prostrate from trying

A woman once came into the surgery and asked me if I would see her husband. 'He's prostrate, Doctor,' she told me behind the back of her hand. I duly went out to see him expecting yet another poor soul fallen to the devil's brew. Instead of a man snoring like something out of *Jurassic Park*, I found a man with a bright red face and crossed legs. He had not passed water for two days and was about to burst at the seams. He was suffering from prostate trouble, and unless the pressure on his bladder was relieved soon, he really would be prostrate, pretty messy too.

If you have found that as time goes by you are unable to push the deodorant blocks down the channel in the urinal, relax. You are in good company. Obstruction of the flow of urine by an enlarged prostate is common, particularly as we get older. Sitting at the neck of the bladder, straddling the tube which carries urine and semen, the prostate is roughly the size of a walnut and has an important job of providing nutrients and protection for the sperm about to make the long journey to the womb. The vagina is a hostile place so far as sperm are concerned; prostatic secretions help neutralise the acid environment found there. Sperm have little room for carrying fuel for energy. The prostate produces large amounts of fructose, an easily absorbed sugar, to keep the engines running. It has nothing to do with the sex drive, which is a shame as the prostate enlarges with age. Should it enlarge too much it can obstruct and even completely halt the flow of urine from the bladder to the penis. When this is caused by simple enlargement with no involvement of cancer, it is referred to as Benign Prostatic Hypertrophy (BPH).

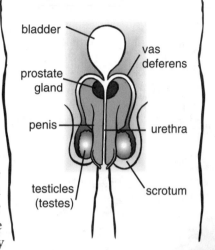

Common problem

Over 30 per cent of men will have some problem with passing urine by the time they reach 50 years of age, yet only half of those men suffering will consult their doctors. Most men put it down to the inevitability of ageing. Many men, as high as 20 per cent of 40 year olds, will need some form of treatment before they die. We don't know why the prostate enlarges but there are certain triggers:

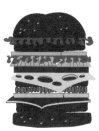

- High levels of testosterone.
- An imbalance between oestrogen and testosterone.
- Possibly low protein, high carbohydrate diets.
- Western diets.

Symptoms of an enlarged prostate

Sure signs of an enlarged prostate are:

- Poor flow.
- Frequent trips to the toilet, even during the night.
- A persistent feeling of 'not quite emptying the bladder', often associated with dribbling after passing urine.
- Traces of blood in urine or in sperm sometimes occur and should always be reported to your doctor.

Your doctor can perform a few simple tests to check the size of your prostate and make sure it is nothing nasty.

Detection

Early detection is vital. The way an enlarged prostate affects you is very important to your doctor. Just from your description alone a working diagnosis can often be made. By examining your rectum, your doctor can check whether your prostate is enlarged. Blood tests will also give some indication of why your prostate is enlarged, as some of the tests are fairly specific for cancer. Ultrasound is also used by passing a sensor into the rectum to visualise the prostate.

Treatment

Happily we are not doomed to walking around with a street map showing all the public conveniences. With modern treatment the outlook is often far from gloomy.

Drugs

A number of medications are available which relax the muscles that are making matters worse. Side effects of the more commonly used drugs include a dry mouth and a slow response from the heart when standing up. This may cause a drop in blood pressure and cause dizziness.

Surgery

If drugs fail or the obstruction becomes complete, surgery is required. What was once a major operation is now simplicity itself. Trans-urethral prostatectomy (TURP) has revolutionised the treatment of enlarged prostates. There are 40,000 prostatectomies of various types performed in the UK each year. Using laser, heat or microwaves, the prostate lobes are trimmed from the inside. It takes about an hour, depending on how much tissue has to be removed, and you will only be in hospital for a day or two. Still under trial are revolutionary new methods which use robots under computer control to guide the tool removing the prostate tissue.

Complications

Some men report a period of impotence after the operation which is usually temporary and is probably psychological rather than a direct effect of surgery. Even so, for the men concerned it is a very real problem and your GP may help with expert counselling. Most effects will wear off within two days. In cases of total impotence, implantable prostheses can be used. 'Retrograde ejaculation', where the sperm are directed into the bladder instead of the penis, often occurs because the one-way valve at the neck of the bladder has to be widened to make effective the operation. It will not cause any pain or harm but it obviously can affect the number of sperm leaving the penis during ejaculation and thus fertility. This complication is not rare but should not affect your enjoyment of sex.

Prostate cancer

Remember, cancer of the prostate can sometimes cause the same symptoms as benign prostatic hypertrophy and be completely painless, but early prostate cancer is almost always symptomless. It will kill over 9,000 men each year in the UK which is four times as many men as cervical cancer will kill women. It mainly affects men between 65 and 70 years, although men as young as 55 can also develop the cancer. Survival at the age of 70 years is 50 per cent. We do not know what causes prostatic cancer, but early diagnosis is essential for successful treatment.

You are more at risk of developing prostate cancer if:

- A close member of your family (brother, father) has developed the cancer.
- You have high levels of testosterone.
- You are Afro-Caribbean.
- You eat a diet rich in animal products, particularly animal fat.
- You are over 70 years of age.

Prevention

It is interesting that men from Japan and China have the lowest rates of prostate cancer in the world and this may be a valuable clue for prevention, particularly as this protection disappears if these men move to areas with a Western diet. The role of dietary oestrogen, and traces of the hormone picked up from pollution, has been shown to be a factor in the stimulation of prostatic cancer. As oestrogen levels may be elevated in obese men, weight reduction is strongly advised. As in many other cancers, antioxidants could be useful in preventing the disease. Vitamins E and C and beta carotene mop up free radicals which damage genetic material in the cells leading to cancer. Zinc is used by the body to make an enzyme which acts like a switch for certain protective genes. Red meat is considered a major factor in stimulating the cancer, while nuts and seeds act as barriers.

A sensible protective diet would involve:

- Reduce all fats; especially limit animal fat intake. It should represent about 25–30 per cent of your energy needs.
- Eat chicken and fish instead of red meat.
- Eat at least half a kilo of fresh fruit per day.
- Take a tip from the Orientals, eat their food.
- Eat nuts and seeds, rather than sweets.
- Increase your intake of antioxidants by eating carrots and citrus fruits, or supplement them in your diet.

Detection

Along with rectal examination, your doctor can perform a blood test for enzymes (acid phosphatase) released by the tumour. A recent development which identifies proteins specific to the cancer (prostate specific antigen) looks promising and may be a means of screening for the disease. Ultrasound is useful but cannot detect very early cancers of the prostate. No matter what method is used, early detection could be the key to successful treatment, so if you are concerned, and particularly if you fall into the higher risk groups, you should think about seeing your doctor.

Treatment

Treatment can involve surgery and radiotherapy to either remove or reduce the bulk of the growth. Regular drug implants under the skin inhibits testosterone from stimulating the growth of the tumour. You will need to use these drugs for the rest of your life. Even if all of the tumour cannot be removed by surgery, this medication can slow it down quite dramatically, giving the man a relatively normal life, many living to a ripe old age and dying from something other than their prostatic cancer.

Unwanted effects of treatment

Side effects depend upon the way the tumour is treated.

- Radiotherapy is used for early cancers or when the tumour cannot be reduced by surgery. It is also very useful in reducing pain, particularly if the tumour has settled in bone. Temporary irritation of the bladder is common with a burning sensation when passing water. On the plus side, radiotherapy may not cause impotence.
- Surgery can damage nerves which control erection, resulting in impotence, but is now less common with improved techniques.
- Hormone treatment can often result in impotence although it is possible to implant a penile prosthesis in some cases. There are also drugs available (papaverine, for example) which cause an erection when injected correctly.

The trouble with gentiles

A man once came
into the surgery
and told me he was
having trouble with
his gentiles. I was
more surprised to
actually see a man come
in to see me with nether
region worries than by
his biblical inexactitude.
Getting men to visit their
doctor for any reason is
difficult at the best of times, and
they are particularly slow to attend with
problems in their boxer shorts, which is a
pity. Many would live a lot longer if they
did, as 95 per cent of all testicular cancers
are successfully treated if caught early.

A whole new ball game

Loosely held in the scrotum, the testes have a number of functions, such as secreting testosterone and developing sperm. After puberty the testes produce sperm at a fairly constant rate. If they are not ejaculated the sperm are reabsorbed. We don't really know why the testes hang outside the body, and most men could think of plenty of less vulnerable places. The fact that sperm production maximises at temperatures slightly lower than that of the body, may offer a reason. On the plus side, having them in such a handy place makes self-examination much easier than if, for instance, they were between your shoulder blades. Few men will dispute the amount of pain which follows a judicious kick in the groin, as testes are well served by nerve fibres. However, serious conditions such as cancer can be quite painless, making regular examination all the more important.

VERY HOT!

HOT

WARM

COOL

COLD

Early death

Of the 1,600 cases reported each year in the UK, around 130 men, often under 30 years old, will die from cancer of the testes. Although it is relatively rare, representing only one per cent of all cancers in men, it is the single biggest cause of cancer-related death in men aged between 18 and 35 years. The number of cases has doubled in the last 20 years and is still rising. We don't know why this is so, but with early recognition of the problem and prompt treatment, few men need to lose their lives.

Cause unknown

As yet we do not know the cause of testicular cancer but research has implicated a number of factors. Young boys are now routinely examined for undescended testes. Boys whose testes have descended normally stand a 1 in 450 chance of developing testicular cancer in later life, while the risk to those whose testes do not descend is increased by a factor of five. It is very important, therefore, to have this condition corrected as early as possible.

Oestrogen has also been identified as a contributing factor. A link has been made between obesity and testicular cancer on the grounds that oestrogen is produced by fatty tissues. It is now thought that some foods, like milk, eaten by mothers during pregnancy could be suspect because they contain oestrogen, and even the safety of water supplies has been called into question, containing, as they do, trace amounts of oestrogen from the contraceptive pill passed in women's urine. Phthalates are also implicated because this plasticiser, found in most plastic food wrappings, can exert an oestrogen-like effect. The unborn male may be adversely affected by these substances without the mother being aware of the risk.

In the family

As with some other cancers, testicular cancer can run in families. If you have a brother who has had this cancer, your chances of developing the condition are ten times greater. This doesn't mean you *will* develop cancer of the testes but you should pay close attention to any changes which may occur in their shape or in how they feel. Evidence from the USA shows that white men have a six times greater incidence of testicular cancer than black men. Similarly, Oriental men also have a lower rate of this disease, as well as a lower rate of prostate cancer.

Being 'testes aware'

Check your testes monthly in the following manner. Do it while lying in a warm bath or while having a long shower, as this makes the skin of the scrotum softer and therefore easier to feel the testes inside.

- Cradle the scrotum in the palm of your hand. Feel the difference between the testes. You will almost definitely feel that one is larger and lying lower. This is completely normal. Ask any tailor.

- Examine each one in turn, and then compare them with each other. Use both hands and gently roll each testicle between thumb and forefinger. Check for any lumps or swellings, as they should both be smooth. Remember that the duct carrying sperm to the penis, the epididymis, normally feels bumpy. It lies along the top and back of the testes.

If you feel anything out of the ordinary, let your GP check them for you. Remember, cancer is often painless, so don't delay. If there is a problem, you will be referred to a specialist. Try not to smile too much when performing the examination; this could give the wrong impression to the person sitting next to you in the railway carriage.

Hospital tests

- You will be glad to hear that you will be physically examined once more. By this time most of the embarrassment has worn off anyway.
- Ultrasound is sometimes used to visualise the testes through the scrotum.
- Blood tests will identify marker proteins such as human chorionic gonadotrophin which are present in much larger amounts in testicular cancer.
- Any spread of the tumour can be located with a CT scan, a sophisticated form of x-ray examination.

Treatment will depend on what is found from these tests, which will exclude simple problems like cysts or infections.

Treatment

You may need the affected testis removed. This will not

necessarily mean that you cannot have children; the remaining testis will produce enough sperm to allow conception. If you had only one testis, or if chemotherapy or radiation is used, it is possible to freeze your sperm and store it. You will not appear strange either. A special implant makes the scrotum look and feel like normal. A single testis is more than adequate to maintain testosterone levels. If both testes are damaged, either from disease or treatment, hormone replacement will supplement your testosterone levels. Impotence is *not* an automatic result of treatment but it can occur in a small number of cases. Sex can still be enjoyed, and most reported problems are psychological rather than physical.

Sensible approach

Obsessive examination and fear can make life miserable. Keep it all in perspective. We only get one chance at life and this one is not a dress rehearsal. Even so, you may be glad you showed your doctor the boxer shorts you got as a Christmas present.

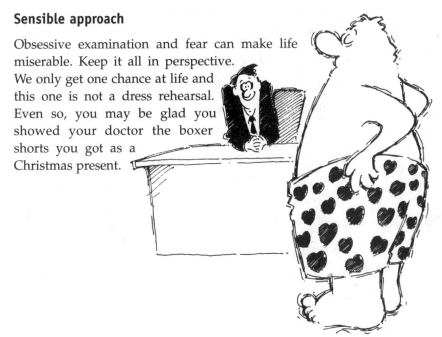

It's a snip – fertility

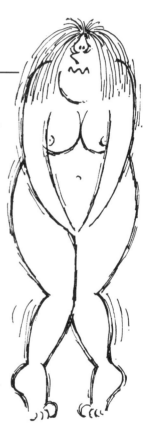

Men have traditionally been the lucky ones when it came to contraception. Throughout history women have not only had to provide contraception but also bear the consequences of failure. This included the use of a primitive 'cap' in the form of a hollowed-out lemon. Now you know why women appear all dewy-eyed in old paintings. Relatively recently, vasectomy for men has shifted the responsibility if not the watery eyes.

Sperm are carried from the testes to the penis by means of two goolie super-highways called the vas deferens (see diagram, page 129). Under local anaesthetic, these can be cut and tied off through a small opening in the scrotum. The operation itself is painless and takes only a few minutes. There can be some discomfort for a few days afterwards. If you are in continual pain, or your scrotum becomes hot and swollen, you should return to your surgeon.

It is effective
Only one vasectomy in 2,500 will spontaneously reverse. However, it is never guaranteed 100 per cent.

It is simple and painless
A number of surgeons with long necks have actually performed their own vasectomies.

It is safe
There have been no reports of any deaths. Plenty of men walking like John Wayne for a few days, but no deaths. There is some concern that testosterone levels can fall in vasectomised men as they grow older. The jury is still out and more evidence is required. Increased cancer of the prostate has also been linked to vasectomy, but studies by the World Health Organisation have found no evidence for this claim.

It is not grief free
Most surgeons will avoid performing the operation on a young childless man. With a divorce rate of one marriage in three, some vasectomised men find themselves in a new relationship with no prospect of children. It is possible to have your

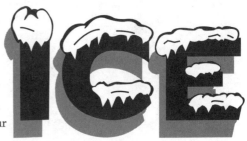

sperm frozen indefinitely, although most clinics prefer them to be used within five years.

After the operation you should wear supportive underpants and avoid lifting heavy weights for a few days. You may resume sex as soon as you feel comfortable but you should use some form of contraception until your sperm count drops to zero. You will be checked for this over a number of weeks.

One in 33 vasectomised men will seek a reversal. They are usually men in their forties who have remarried a childless younger woman. It is possible to have the reversal performed on the NHS but waiting lists tend to be long as it is a common operation. It will cost you around £1,200 to have your privates treated privately. The success rate is far from 100 per cent and depends upon many factors, not least the way the vasectomy was performed in the first place. In some cases antibodies to sperm are produced after vasectomy which inhibit them from swimming properly.

If you find vasectomies too complicated I still have those two house bricks in my bottom drawer. Call anytime, bring a box of tissues.

Out for the count

Long, long ago a man containing a large amount of falling-down water came into casualty at three in the morning demanding a sperm count. A young, tired but good-looking casualty officer gave him a milk bottle and told him to come back when it was full.

A recent report in the *British Medical Journal* highlighted the decline in quality and quantity of sperm throughout Europe. Men born after around 1970 have a disturbingly high number of abnormal sperm. Basically sperm are tiny torpedoes with a warhead full of genetic material, DNA, an engine and a propeller in the form of a tail. Although millions of sperm are released with each ejaculation, relatively few ever reach the egg, and only one will actually fertilise it. Abnormal sperm can be seen through the microscope as having two heads, two tails, or headless, or tail-less. Despite looking perfectly normal, some sperm appear unable to swim at all. As the number of normal sperm falls so the chances of successful conception are reduced. While there are enormous numbers being produced it doesn't really matter, but below a certain point the man is said to have impaired fertility.

Worryingly the article points out a 2 per cent decline each year in the number of sperm men produce. Predictions are that men in the new millennium may be unable to produce any normal sperm, with obvious consequences for the human race. The article blames plastics, pollution and oestrogen in recycled water which may be affecting the unborn male child and could explain the dramatic two-fold increase in undescended testes and testicular cancer over the past 20 years (see page 136). Worse still, there may be a link with the increasing numbers of babies born with both male and female genitalia.

Tight trousers and driving for too long are both possible causes in the reduced production of normal sperm. This is probably due to constant warming of the testes, which prefer a cooler than body temperature for maximal sperm production.

It can be very distressing for a man to be told he has abnormal and reduced numbers of sperm. There is no cure for this problem but it doesn't always mean that having children is impossible. Healthy sperm can be separated out and given a short cut by placing them directly into the cervix. In vitro fertilisation (IVF) is now almost routine, where sperm and egg are brought together in the laboratory before being returned to the womb.

Nevertheless the trend is causing much concern. It is just our luck not only to suffer more from every medical condition common to both sexes but we are also being attacked where it hurts most. It is going to take a seriously high degree of action from the government to address and reverse the problem.

After all this you won't be surprised to hear that the man who was given the milk bottle in the wee small hours never came back.

Male hormone replacement therapy

When one of my patients walked in and said, 'I need a patch, Doc', I thought he had a sore eye. Not so. It transpired that he had read a newspaper report extolling the virtues of Hormone Replacement Therapy (HRT) for men. Despite controversy and early claims that proved to be too optimistic, HRT for women has a lot going for it, especially in the prevention of osteoporosis, the thinning of the bones. Now, perhaps, men too can benefit from

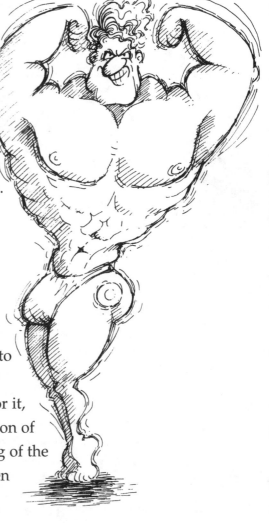

similar therapy. In the USA a patch has been developed which gradually releases testosterone, the male sex hormone, and it is available in the UK.

The media have reported enthusiastically on the beneficial effects this treatment can have on libido, muscle development and general wellbeing, but most of the information comes from a sensationalist and ill-informed press. When things are not going quite right in the sex department, or at work or within the family, it is tempting to look for a simple cause and lack of testosterone is an easy target. Even though it may not be quite the wonder drug claimed by some, HRT (or more accurately TRT – Testosterone Replacement Therapy) has become a real possibility for men and will enhance their lives.

Role of testosterone

Testosterone is released from the testes under direct control of the pituitary, a small gland in the brain. This gland secretes follicle stimulating hormone, FSH, which stimulates the production of sperm and luteinising hormone, LH, which stimulates the testes to produce testosterone. It is partly responsible for secondary male characteristics such as facial hair, and also has a role in maintaining muscle power and keeps your tackle in good order. If you lose your testes before

MUSCLE

puberty, your voice will not lower in pitch and you will keep a full head of hair. Testosterone is important in the development of bone, and lack of it can cause thinning of the bones leading to easy fracture. Blood levels of testosterone remain fairly steady with a gradual fall over the years. For some unknown reason testosterone exerts a diminishing effect as we get older but big falls in blood levels only occur with damage or disease of either the pituitary or testes. Men with hypogonadism have a reduction in the amount of testosterone in their blood. Muscle mass decreases, their bones can thin and they often suffer a general feeling of tiredness all the time. Hormone replacement for these men is essential to maintain normal body functions. The manufacture of testosterone hormone replacement means that deficiencies in testosterone can be made good.

Penile erectile dysfunction

Most men who request hormone replacement therapy do so in the hope of correcting their penile erectile dysfunction, or impotence. This is a common problem, but except for recognised medical conditions such as advanced diabetes, there is often no organic reason for its occurrence. In fact, levels of testosterone are usually normal in men with erectile dysfunction. Sexual problems, stress, tiredness or marital disharmony are more commonly the main culprits.

Building hormone

Testosterone's involvement in building muscles has been exploited by men obsessed with body building. Earlier forms of testosterone were dangerous in high doses and have been withdrawn in the UK. Injections of high doses of testosterone may increase muscle mass but they can also have serious side effects on the heart and liver. Short-term gains of bulging muscles are a poor recompense for a weakened heart and a failing liver. It only makes you a healthy-looking corpse.

Danger

Some cancers are stimulated to grow by hormones. Prostate cancer thrives on testosterone. In fact, by stopping the body producing testosterone, the tumour's growth often slows down. Giving high doses of testosterone to a man with undiagnosed prostate cancer could be clearly disastrous, so he must first be carefully checked. A rectal examination gives some indication of any problems that may be present but blood tests are more accurate (see pages 132–4).

The male menopause

At a certain stage in a man's life, usually around 45 to 55 years of age, a so-called mid-life crisis can occur. It has been labelled the 'male menopause' or the 'viropause', although there is little comparison to the female menopause. Unlike women, there is no evidence of a dramatic drop in sex hormone levels. However, some researchers have argued that the reason why we don't have any evidence of hormonal variation in men is because we are looking at the wrong hormones. They suggest that instead of testosterone, the hormones FSH and LH should be measured. Measurement should also be made of the protein SHBG, sex hormone binding globulin, which attaches to testosterone as it circulates in the blood, rendering the hormone inactive until released. The levels of bound testosterone gradually rise with age, thus reducing the effects of testosterone on the target organs.

We do know that it is at this time of life that uncertainty, underconfidence and inability to fit the media image of a sexually powerful, competitive macho male can affect a man's self-esteem. Compounding all this is the fear of ageing. It is tempting to simply put this crisis down to a lack of sex hormone, and some of the claims for testosterone therapy go beyond what can be achieved by replacing what is missing, which in turn can be too eagerly accepted by men with no organic problems.

Many things have an effect on testosterone levels. Chronic alcohol abuse, for instance, reduces the ability of the testes to produce testosterone. If you think you would benefit from TRT, get it clear in your mind *why* you would like it and then sit down with your doctor. Most of the problems people hope to be 'cured' by TRT can be solved without any hormone treatment. Check it out:

- Sort out problems with your partner; counselling can help.
- Take a close look at your life style and see if you are smoking, drinking or avoiding exercise. These will all contribute to a vicious circle of feel-bad factors.
- Ditch that beer gut. Only people like dart players get away with it anyway.
- Relax, rather than collapse. You can be active and yet relax. Kids are a marvellous source of cheap entertainment and relaxation, if you are prepared to be

the horse/elephant/train.

- On the other hand get rid of the kids. Not necessarily to the local white slaver, but sex and intimacy can improve when the children are with someone else for the night. A romantic break can be as simple as telling the kids to entertain themselves for a couple of hours while you have a cuddle. Better still, take a night away once in a while and let the in-laws benefit from all the exercise of being a horse/elephant/train for a change.

- Hypogonadism (clinical deficiencies of testosterone) is rare. It is estimated that only 20,000 men will suffer from it in the UK. That's less than one man per general practitioner.

- Menopause is a strictly female phenomenon as men do not have a menses (period). Viropause and andropause are the so-called equivalents for men but their existence is hotly disputed by leading endocrinologists (doctors dealing with hormones).

- Cancer of the pituitary can mimic a problem with the testes by failing to stimulate them to produce testosterone. This needs to be checked before any therapy.

- Testosterone stimulates the growth of an established prostate cancer. There is as yet no definitive test for prostate cancer but the presence of prostate specific antigen and a rectal examination come very close. Even so you should be checked every six months while on TRT.

The pain drain

A patient once walked into
casualty and
asked me did I
have anything
for pain, so I
showed him
what we use for
removing tonsils. 'This
should make your eyes
water,' I told him. The
brain truly is a marvellous
invention. Not only does it
keep your ears apart so you can
really appreciate Oasis in stereo,
it also tells you when you need
to look for your fingertips in
the mince.

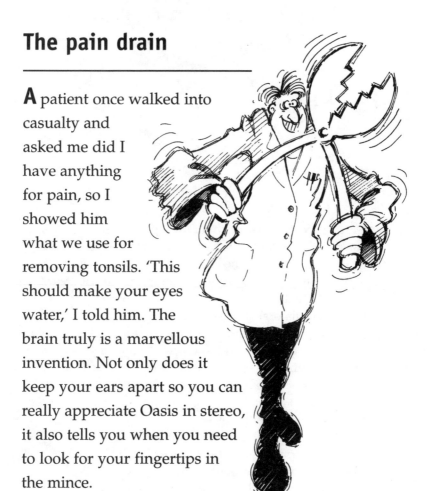

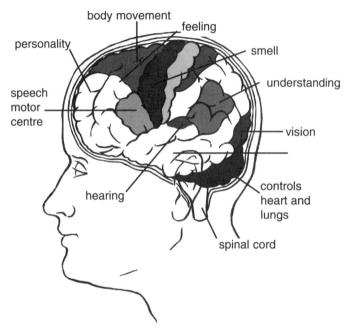

Despite the fact that the brain cannot 'feel' pain itself as it has no pain sensors, it has a sophisticated system of recognising pain. All over the body tiny sensors detect pressure, temperature and pain. They are not evenly distributed. Use a pair of dividers (the ones in a school geometry kit not two pocket calculators) to see how close together you can put the points and still tell they are two separate jags when you place them on your skin. The tips of your fingers or your lips are much more sensitive than say, your back. It is probably best not to test your eyes with this device and I would take it as read that a certain other part of your body is pretty sensitive as well.

Touching something very hot will provoke a rapid withdrawal reaction. This reflex arc skips the brain and only uses the spinal cord to stimulate the muscles. Strangely enough you can provoke a similar reflex action by tapping a stretched tendon, such as at the bent knee. Hence the term, 'testing your reflexes'. I have the same reflex action when any of my kids touch something very expensive in a toy shop. This is called 'reflexes by proxy' and is present in all parents.

Once a pain sensor has been stimulated, the signal is sent along peripheral nerve fibres to the spinal cord. It has to cross a number of junctions, synapses, between nerves before the signal gets to the brain. By inserting a vibrating needle, or stimulating the nerve with a mild electric current, this transfer can be blocked and the sensation of pain is diminished. This partly explains how acupuncture and TENS (transcutaneous electrical neural stimulation) work. Alternatively, injections of local anaesthetic around the spinal cord, an epidural, will stop any signals moving past this point. Unfortunately it also makes your legs think it is Friday night.

Once it has reached the brain, pain is subject to all kinds of modification. Agony in one set of circumstances can become ecstasy in another. Some pain is held at bay until the brain decides it needs some attention. Rugby players have been known to break their arms without realising it until someone shakes their hand at the end of the match. Hypnosis and distraction work at this level. If you hit yourself in the groin with a hammer, it will quite nicely take your mind off the ingrowing toenail on your big toe. That is why they are called ball-peen hammers.

Headache

People frequently suffer from headaches and tension is probably the most common cause. In these circumstances, fretting that your headache is caused by something more serious will only make matters worse. Relaxation techniques can sometimes work wonders for headaches resistant to the strongest painkillers.

One of the worst things about a headache is that no one can see the pain. You need to screw your face up and peer through half-closed eyes before anyone is impressed. Some headaches still won't attract sympathy no matter how much you make a face. Self-inflicted varieties are more likely to result in a short lecture on the dangers of alcohol abuse. Rehydration, vitamin c and paracetamol usually help.

Migraine is common and runs in families. Certain foods appear to trigger an attack. Red wine, particularly Chianti, blue cheeses and chocolate are all culprits. Stress, the weather and even hormone changes have been known to increase the suffering. Visual patterns like chequerboards are often a warning of an impending attack. Light can hurt the eyes and lying in a darkened room can help some people. The attack can last from minutes to days. A specific migraine therapy, Imigran injections or tablets may reduce or even prevent a full-blown migraine attack, when given or taken early in an attack. Several other treatments (such as beta-blockers) can be taken regularly to reduce the number of attacks.

Sinusitis is nasty. Infection of the spaces in the facial bones causes a pain worse on stooping or pooping. Antibiotics are usually the answer.

Meningitis is a different kettle of fish. To some extent it can mimic a migraine attack or even a simple headache. Symptoms usually come on very rapidly, so you need to be alert to the possibility of this dreadful disease. Temperature will usually be raised, and vomiting is common. A blue-black rash, often over the buttocks, tends to appear later in the course of the illness. Light, even daylight, can be agony and this photophobia is a warning that all is not well. Increasing drowsiness and lethargy are frequent signs. Confusion, slurred speech and poor balance may be present. In children, all or none of these symptoms may be present and a child may simply be suddenly unable to walk or talk. Time is all important. With early diagnosis meningitis can be cured without any brain damage. If you are not sure what is happening give your doctor a ring, otherwise go to casualty immediately, where the child will be given antibiotics.

Despite being rare, brain tumours are on the increase amongst young adults. In the search for a cause certain pollutants are under investigation. Successful treatment depends on the type of tumour and its location. Tragically they may not make their presence felt until too late. Persistent vomiting is often an early indication of rising pressure within the skull; double vision and poor balance can also occur. Depending upon where the tumour lies, specific functions can be affected. A tumour at the auditory nerve, for instance, can cause deafness on that side. Sometimes the only indication that a tumour exists will be a subtle change in taste or smell.

Headaches are common and fortunately serious causes are rare.

Getting the better of stress

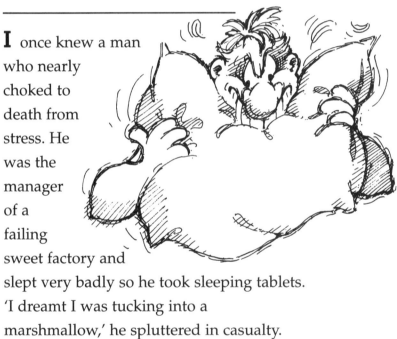

I once knew a man
who nearly
choked to
death from
stress. He
was the
manager
of a
failing
sweet factory and
slept very badly so he took sleeping tablets.
'I dreamt I was tucking into a
marshmallow,' he spluttered in casualty.
'When I woke up I was eating the pillow.'
His wife was only glad he wasn't dreaming
of jelly babies.

Some people thrive on the 'stress' of the job and use it to produce an excellent performance. Actors, for instance, will often speak of their need for the rush of adrenaline to peak. Adrenaline is called the fight or flight hormone as it readies the body for action:

- Blood sugar goes up to supply energy.
- The bowels empty and the blood supply goes down.
- The pupils of the eyes dilate.
- Heart rate and blood pressure rise along with breathing more deeply.

It is when this normal reaction is not allowed to release itself (in fight or flight) and remains a constant state that stress can be harmful. Perhaps surprisingly, unemployment or job insecurity causes more stress-related illness than having stable permanent work no matter how demanding.

As stress builds up there is a recognised pattern of behaviour:

- Constant fatigue and poor sleep patterns.
- Poor concentration and short-term memory; it is difficult to follow a long conversation.
- Introspection increases. Only matters of direct relevance to the stress factors, earning money, travel, etc., appear important.
- Personal and family neglect: personal appearance becomes irrelevant; children and partners become obstructions to, rather than assets for, pleasure.
- Repetitive behaviour is common. You will find yourself constantly going round the house switching off lights or checking the hot tap hourly for drips.
- Alcohol or even drugs can be abused, particularly to get some sleep or relaxation.
- Irritability increases, a short fuse develops where very little will spark off a reaction. Don't ask me why. It just does, cos I said so, OK? Wanna make something of it?

Easy to give advice

It can be difficult to act upon good advice even when it is obvious that a problem is building up. This may be due to financial, social or personal pressures. However, there may also be a failure to recognise and defuse stress triggers before they begin to cause all the difficulties. Late trains, late milkmen, even late relations can cause stress. Barking dogs, smokers in no-smoking areas, traffic jams, long queues at the checkout, the list is endless. These will not go away, but recognising them as stress triggers and coping with them is halfway to reducing their effects.

Stress triggers

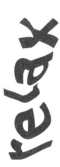

Remember your stress triggers and when you get caught up in one, use it as a cue to relax. When minor things occur which would normally annoy and stress you – engaged phones, the bus that sails on past your out-stretched arm – recognise that these are all trivia. Watch how other people react, some will stamp and curse over so little, while others will give a sideways grin. Who will live longer?

Do's and don'ts

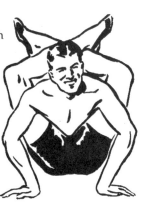

- Exercise is an excellent way to burn off frustration and stress. Sport which appears stressful can often be the opposite. Or try peaceful and gentle relaxation techniques such as yoga. Both ways of reducing stress will help sleep patterns without the need to resort to drugs or alcohol.
- Alcohol and smoking will, at best, provide only short-term relief from the effects of stress. At their very worst, in excess, they will

produce their own problems which will make whatever was previously causing your stress seem like a holiday. Ask someone who has had a heart attack. Their life is suddenly thrown into perspective and trivia is recognised for what it is.

- You only have one pair of hands. Take jobs in their order of importance instead of trying to do everything at once. Learn to say NO to more work.
- Conversations require give and take. Stop talking *at* people and listen to what they are saying even if it doesn't seem to fit in with all your worries. Play with the kids, it is good exercise and they will love it. Might even tire them out for bedtime, you too.
- Food is important. Eat it, don't just consume it. Chat to people around the table, this is the time to talk about the good things.
- Share a long bath with your partner. Dream and plan holidays.

Loss of job, loss of self-esteem

Being made redundant or losing a job is a major life event; it is significant that suicide in young men rose by 75 per cent between 1982 and 1991. Instability of work may well have been a factor. Even retirement can cause depression, particularly in men. There is an increase in depression immediately following retirement which, if not corrected, can rumble on making life miserable for both the man and his partner. Restoration of the feeling of self-worth is fundamental to many such problems.

GPs are specially trained to recognise and treat depression. They are a natural source of help as they will know you and your family yet will respect your need for confidentiality. Treating depression is as much a part of their everyday work as treating high blood pressure, so don't feel you are wasting their time. It's surprising how much can be done once you share the load with someone who knows just how to deal with these problems.

Antidepressant medications are usually well tolerated, are non-addictive and are commonly prescribed for three to six months or even longer. Tranquillisers, such as diazepam, can provide short-term relief in anxiety, but can cause addiction if taken for periods longer than as little as four to six weeks. Modern trends in the treatment of stress, on the other hand, avoid the use of drugs, concentrating instead on the cause. Diet can be important. Vitamin B complexes and vitamin C are badly depleted in chronic stress. This is made worse if you resort to alcohol as it makes the levels even lower. Buy a pet. Studies have shown that men with pets live longer than those without. Choose your pet with care. Piranha fish can be difficult to stroke with finger stumps.

Diversionary tactics

It is very easy to say 'relax' but like many pieces of advice, it can be harder to practise than to preach. Simply saying 'I will relax' can lead to a cycle of even worse tension. Distraction can help.

- Look around you. How many people passing you have blond hair? What is the commonest hairstyle? How many women are wearing mini skirts? You can choose your own distraction but try not to select something which will only reinforce your anxiety, like how many dentists' surgeries you pass on the way to have a tooth extracted.

- Physical activity can be a marvellous release of tension. Almost any physical effort will work, painting, walking, sport or aerobics.
- Mental activity, so long as it is not related to the cause of your anxiety, will also help. If your source of anxiety is the forthcoming dental appointment, try reading a funny book rather than *Marathon Man*.

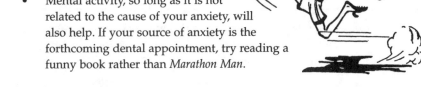

Relaxation exercises

Reading a book on how to play the piano will not turn you into a concert pianist. Practice makes perfect, and this applies to learning how to relax without resorting to alcohol or drugs. As you become proficient in relaxation you will find you do not need formal, structured exercises but can do the job almost unconsciously. Like playing the piano 'instinctively', there can be a long period of training.

Make sure you will be alone; it will not help if you are constantly disturbed by requests for another drink of water or to answer a telephone. Either lie on a bed or sit in a chair with your head and arms supported and feet on a stool. Settle down and rid your mind of any thoughts which increase your anxiety – concentrate on the positive words such as 'relax' or 'unwind'. Gentle music may help but is not essential. Breathe in deeply and hold your breath. Gradually release your breath and, as you do so, let your body sink into the chair or bed.

Focusing your tension and release into specific parts of your body can be very effective. Concentrate on your right hand, make it into a fist, tightly clench it, then release it. Do it again. This time concentrate on the tension in your hand and as you release it notice the difference in the way it feels from when it is clenched and when it is relaxed. Do the same with your arms. Flex them and feel the tension build up as you bend your elbow. Imagine you are pulling a heavy weight. Hold the tension for a while and then relax. As you relax breathe out. At the same time reinforce the relaxation by thinking positive thoughts, 'I feel better', 'I am relaxing'. By concentrating on the difference between the relaxed and tensed state of your muscles and linking it to your mental state, there will be a logical sequence of reinforcement. Use a set pattern:

- After tensing a muscle always return to a relaxed state.
- Do you feel the effect? Concentrate on the difference.
- Use a pattern for breathing. Always breathe in as you tense your muscles and breathe out as you relax.
- Even if you think you have completely relaxed a muscle, try to release it that bit more.
- Take your time. It will become easier to achieve a state of relaxation more quickly as you become more adept.
- Use positive thoughts to augment your physical activity, 'relax', 'let go', etc.
- Repeat each individual exercise at least twice. You will be surprised at the level of relaxation you will achieve after each repeat.
- Use the same pathway for each part of your body – neck, chest, abdomen, legs, feet, and so on. You do not have to adhere rigidly to this system; you will soon find a pattern which suits you best.

Now is the time to reflect both on the trivia which can cause such tension and how, with a little practice, they can be seen in their true light. On the other hand, you might still feel like pulling all your hair out by the roots, but at least you won't get out of breath.

Down in the dumps

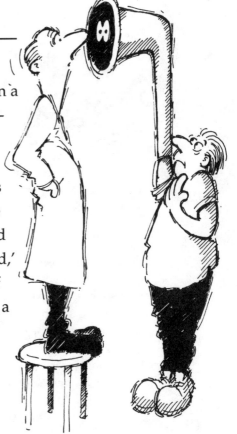

A man once came into casualty with his arm stuck in a length of four-inch conduit U-bend. 'I feel depressed,' he told me, as I called for the fire brigade. As he waved his arm around like a submarine periscope, I could understand his predicament. 'Never mind,' says I, trying that old ploy of humour guaranteed to bring a smile even to the face of a dying man. 'At least it's not stuck on some other part of your anatomy.' With a sigh reminiscent of a deflating poopie cushion, he replied, 'That's what I am depressed about. That's why my arm is stuck in this here pipe.' Despite all my training and experience as a doctor, I still wonder to this day what he meant.

Suffering from depression is not the same as suffering from stress. Depression is caused by an imbalance of hormones within the brain. For example serotonin, a neurotransmitter, is produced in lower amounts. We don't know why this happens but almost one in six people suffer from a mental health problem. Figures for 1995 from the British Office of Population Censuses and Surveys show that out of a total of 10,000 adults 16 per cent had a psychotic or neurotic disorder of some kind.

A scale of misery

The most common age for any form of depressive illness in men is around 50–66 years, with many cases going undiagnosed. There are two types of depression, although there is often some degree of overlap.

Reactive depression

Reactive depression is a consequence, a reaction to what is happening to you. If you have just lost your job or your partner has left you and has taken the lottery ticket with them, it is a safe bet that you will feel depressed. Life events are given a scale of impact. For instance, death of a partner or child comes very high on the list, and moving house is surprisingly very far up the scale. Although many men will turn up at the doctor's surgery for medicines, there is actually very little that drugs will do to help this type of depression. Only by changing your circumstances will you be able to lift your mental state. Men have little opportunity to express their emotions as do women and tend to build it all up inside them. Groups like the Samaritans are experts in helping men through the rocky times such as divorce.

Endogenous depression

Endogenous depression is another thing altogether. Despite having just won on the lottery and been promoted to the top job, you still feel depressed. This type of depression can be inherited, affecting successive generations in a family. Depression can have a whole battery of effects:

- Weight loss
- Poor sleep patterns
- Early waking
- Reduced appetite
- Reduced libido
- High emotional state. Bursting into tears is common.
- Poor self-confidence
- Poor self-image
- Thoughts of self-harm and suicide

Eating

Eating stimulates a pleasure sensor in the brain releasing a group of hormones called endorphins. These hormones produce the feeling of wellbeing and contentment often experienced after a meal. For whatever reason, depression reduces the desire for food, itself a powerful survival factor. Agitation with poor sleep patterns serve only to burn up more calories than usual, which are not being replaced and weight loss is inevitable and rapid. A vicious circle is then set up, with exhaustion and weakness fuelling the depression. It can be difficult to impress on a person in the depths of depression the need to eat.

Poor sleep patterns

The inability to sleep, particularly with early wakening, is a common feature of depression, and can be one of its early manifestations. Many men will visit their GP because of poor sleep and ask for sleeping tablets, which certainly work in the short-term, but quite soon increasingly heavier doses will be needed to induce sleep.

Numerous studies confirm the importance of sleep for normal bodily function. Without a correct pattern of sleep a man may rapidly develop all the symptoms of paranoia, irritability and an inability to cope. Sleeplessness simply adds to the misery of depression. The brain is very active during certain periods of sleep, and REM sleep, vital for normal brain function, is characterised by rapid eye movements. Dreaming is intense at this time and the brain sorts out problems and effectively reduces tension. Sleep which is devoid of REM is often not refreshing and the person wakes feeling as though they have not really slept. Most sleeping tablets reduce the amount of REM sleep as does alcohol. You may have found that although you slept all night after a bout of heavy drinking, you still felt tired in the morning. A second sleep in the late morning or afternoon is far more refreshing as the alcohol has been broken down or washed out of the system. If you are depressed, alcohol abuse is tempting because it blocks out the constant train of unpleasant thoughts. But the tiredness and exhaustion it produces from the lack of REM sleep only makes the next day worse. Many men will spend long periods in bed, not only to avoid contact with other people and having to confront problems, but also to make up for poor sleep patterns.

Reduction in libido

One of the early casualties of depression is sexual drive,

which in a healthy man is a powerful and deep-seated emotion. It ensures the survival of the species, so it is often referred to as an 'ancient' part of brain function. In evolutionary terms, we probably thought about sex long before we considered Life the Universe and Everything. Like the desire to eat, sex takes a low priority during depression. Partly this is due to exhaustion and malnutrition. But animals which have been starved often maintain their sexual drive, and there is even evidence that this can be increased possibly as an evolutionary survival instinct. However, in men suffering from depression, libido usually declines causing friction between partners. Instead of realising that the lack of interest is a symptom of depression, the partner can incorrectly attribute it as its cause. Men themselves who suffer from depression can make exactly the same mistake and visit their GP for sex counselling only to find that depression is the real culprit. Needless to say, the unhappiness and marital disharmony which often results from this friction only serves to enhance the sense of misery during depression. Successful treatment of the underlying depression often restores normal service in this department.

Emotional changes

Fatigue takes its toll on emotion. A constant tiredness makes most people emotionally volatile. If you add depression, the result is a man who can burst into tears with little provocation. Men are not expected by our society to show such emotion and it can be interpreted as a weakness. A depressed man may find coping increasingly difficult and this enhances the impression of a 'lack of manliness'. Far from sympathising and giving support, many employers and relatives will resort to the why-don't-you-pull-yourself-together routine, which is guaranteed to up the pressure and make things even worse. Some men find themselves weeping for no apparent reason. Others find that a relatively minor stimulus such as a television programme or an unguarded word from a colleague will reduce them to tears. Instead of stifling this response, it is better to let it run its course. Many men will wait until they are alone or in bed before releasing this pent-up emotion.

Poor self-image and confidence

Another early casualty is self-image and confidence. Men may suddenly find themselves unable to make a decision. This can happen over simple things like what to eat as well as major, even life-threatening, decisions. One GP who suffered from depression told of working in his practice for three weeks while convinced he was on holiday in France. It was only when his patients complained to his colleagues that they never received any medication did they realise he was in acute depression. Closely related to poor self-confidence is altered self-image. Lack of self-worth is common. Not only do you feel useless, you are convinced that you look pretty useless as well. Sexual attractiveness is often a target for self-deprecation. Along with this comes a declining interest in appearance and hygiene. Not surprisingly, it all becomes a self-fulfilling prophecy. Suicide is now the second greatest cause of death in young men. Recently bereaved men or those recently retired are at risk from self-harm. Seek help from your GP and friends; they can help make you realise that life is worth living after all.

ça va ?

The cavalry is just over the hill

Your GP can help and there is good advice from many organisations. Endogenous depression often responds well to therapy and medication.

- Psychotherapy, a specialised form of counselling, enables a depressed man to talk about his feelings and concerns. It is a useful way of exploring reasons for his depression.
- Antidepressants often work well but take about three weeks to take effect. They should not be stopped abruptly and treatment will continue for a month or so after any improvement has been achieved.
- Electroconvulsive therapy (ECT) is not used as much today as in the past. It is reserved for severe depression which is not responding to other treatments. A small electrical current passed through the skull while anaesthetised induces a convulsion which can have life-saving effects on depression. It is poorly understood by the public at large, however, and receives a bad press.

It is possible to help yourself to moderate the effects of endogenous depression.

- Try to talk about your concerns with a friend or relative who sympathises but is also constructive.
- Regular physical activity helps release pent-up emotions and keeps you fit to cope with the depression.
- Eat food which will keep up your energy, even if you don't feel hungry.
- Avoid using alcohol as a relaxant. It only makes things worse.
- Make a simple plan for the next day before going to sleep. The decision to make a certain phone call or buy a certain food is important. It helps you look ahead.

Healthy and gay

Disease has little concern for a man's sexual orientation. Life can be difficult for young men who are gay or unsure about their sexuality. Many feel isolated, driven by society, school, relatives and even the law. Some can become desperately lonely and depressed. Indeed, the suicide rate is higher among gay teenagers. For most men the process of coming out is a difficult decision, but many are pleasantly surprised by the reception they receive from friends and family. If you are not sure what to do, talk to someone you trust, a friend, teacher or parent. You can also call Friend Helpline on 0171 837 3337

GPs

If you are not on a GP's list, you should register now. Ask your friends for recommendations, it is usually very obvious which GPs make a special effort or are gay themselves. If you are registered and feel that your GP is not approachable over gay issues, choose another one who you know to be better socially adjusted. Ask your local genito-urinary clinic or HIV unit. They will tell you which GPs in the area are 'gay friendly'.

Anal sex

Anal sex is practised by many gay and straight men. Indeed it is a common form of 'contraception' in some cultures. Regular anal sex frequently leads to tiny cuts inside the rectum which has a relatively thin lining. These cuts will often bleed, particularly during anal sex. It is essential, therefore, to take precautions and use a strong condom such as Durex Extra Safe, Mates Extra Strong, HT Specials or Gay Safe. This will protect both you and your partner.

Although extra lubrication is often required, do not use an oil-based lubricant such as Vaseline, baby oil, margarine or butter. They will damage the condom. Use water-based lubricants like KY Jelly or Foreplay. If you are not sure, ask the chemist; they sell thousands of them and will not be embarrassed to give advice.

HIV test

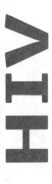

The decision to have a test for HIV infection is a difficult challenge for many gay men. You cannot tell who is HIV positive simply from the way people dress, act or speak, and every time you have unsafe sex you put yourself at risk. In the past many gay men did not ask for a test. They were afraid of insurance companies, building societies and employers discriminating against them. To a very large extent this prejudice has eased.

If you are aware of your HIV status you can adopt a life style which will help keep you healthy. This includes avoiding unnecessary risks to your health and provides your doctor with the insight to recognise more quickly early warning signs of potential medical problems and deal with them more effectively.

It remains a difficult decision, however, and you should discuss it with your friends, partner and doctor. Most centres have good counselling for pre- and post-testing. It is important to remember that the test may give a HIV negative result for up to three months after you have actually become infected. You can pass on the virus to your partner during this time.

Living with HIV

Human Immunodeficiency Virus is a relative newcomer in the medical world, having only been discovered in the early eighties. Although we know a great deal about how it infects and what it does to a person, we have yet to produce a vaccine or a cure, so prevention is the name of the game. People tend to use the terms HIV positive and AIDS interchangeably. This is incorrect. Only when the immune system of an HIV positive person has broken down can they be said to have the Acquired Immune Deficiency Syndrome associated with HIV. Once the body is unable to fight off infections the person is prone to attack from bugs not normally considered a risk to life. This state of affairs has a variable onset but averages out at about 12 years after becoming HIV positive. Survival after developing AIDS is also variable but generally you have a 50 per cent chance of living for three years.

Sounds bad, but things are improving and new vaccines and treatments are just round the corner. Just as well. At the last count over 20,000 people in the UK were HIV positive with over 8,000 suffering from AIDS itself. Most of these are men. The figures may not be accurate as many men do not know their HIV status and some estimates go as high as 40,000 cases in the UK. So should AIDS victims just give up? Not at all. By watching what you eat and drink this survival time can be increased significantly. Most health advice also applies to men with HIV. Avoiding smoking and excess alcohol, for instance, makes good sense. There are some specific points which should be considered.

Diet

Healthy diets are not quite the same when you are HIV positive. Reducing cholesterol and fat intake will reduce your chances of having an early heart attack at, say, 60 years. Common sense will prevail over how useful this diet will be to an HIV-infected man, depending upon his age on infection. In fact, full fat milk, cheeses, creamy yoghurt, butter and ice cream are all preferable to their low fat alternatives. Fat supplies not only a valuable energy source but also vitamins which are only found in fatty products. The ideal body weight for a man with HIV is about 5 kg (11 lb) heavier than for other people of the same height. It is better to be a little overweight than underweight, although frank obesity should be avoided.

Salads are potentially hazardous because they may contain organisms which are potentially dangerous to people with HIV. All vegetables should be thoroughly washed and salads should be avoided outside of your own home or when you cannot be sure if they have been suitably prepared. Chicken, eggs and seafood must be fresh, hygienically stored and thoroughly cooked. Similarly, water, whether from taps or bottled, can also be dangerous. Drink only water that has been boiled then stored in the fridge.

Keeping fit makes good sense for any man, but

HIV men should avoid overexertion. Vaccinations are important, although your GP will advise you on ones which should be omitted. Flu jabs are very important and you should visit your GP each year before the winter.

Doom and gloom

It is easy to see all this as restrictive, but remember you have as much right to happiness as the next man. There is no reason why you should not be sexually active, given the precautions of safer sex. You have a right to be loved and to love. The person you loved before he had the infection is still the same person after the diagnosis, only more precious. Count the do's as well as the don'ts; they usually outnumber them and are more fun anyway. The aim is to be as healthy and happy as possible for as long as possible. So what's new, HIV or no HIV?

First aid

Accidents are
now the single
most common
cause of death
for young men.
We manage to
mangle our Minis, leap
off ladders and hit
very hard things while travelling at high
speeds four times more often than women
do. Sports injuries, industrial accidents and
death from dodgy DIY is our forte. Give the
average man a vari-speed hammer drill and
he won't be content until he has drilled a
hole in his left eyeball. Luckily there are
others around to pick up the pieces. For
every professional medic there are 40 first-
aiders. Which is good news for the guy
about to discover his brake pipes leak.

Myths of first aid

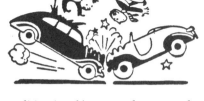

You can be sued if you look after someone and they think you were negligent.

Wrong

The Good Samaritan principle keeps you safe from litigation. You are only expected to be able to do what any other non-medically trained person could do. Carrying out a roadside brain transplant will tend to strain this rule somewhat.

First aid is not really important. Getting them to hospital takes precedence.

Wrong

It is vital to get professional help as soon as possible but ambulance drivers generally like to pick up live people on the way to casualty. A person can lose all their blood from a serious wound in a horribly short space of time. Some jobs need to be done immediately.

Men should not look after injured women in case they are accused of sexual harassment.

Wrong

Common sense prevails. Do what you need to do to save her life. If another woman is present, use her to chaperone. Don't go alone into a toilet with a woman who is confused. Explain out loud what you are doing even if she appears unconscious; it also helps to calm onlookers. While there may undoubtedly be some things worse than death, she is unlikely to be thinking of them while her arm is hanging off.

Doing something is always better than doing nothing.

Wrong

People with absolutely no idea can be a danger to your health. Giving a badly injured person a wee dram might bring their colour back but it only produces a healthy-looking corpse. Even with the most basic insight you will avoid most of these 'first aid' practices, otherwise called euthanasia.

People always faint when they see blood.
Wrong
If you know what you need to do and you get on with it, you
will probably not faint. Onlooking voyeurs usually pass out
in droves, I'm pleased to say. Mind you, black
pudding never tastes the same again.

*You will catch HIV if you perform mouth-to-mouth
resuscitation on someone with AIDS.*
Wrong
Although there is a small theoretical risk, actually you have
more chance of winning the jackpot on the lottery, without
buying a ticket in the first place. You may, however, lose
any passion for garlic or carrots. On the plus side,
you will never buy a drink again at the same bar
as the man you saved.

A little knowledge is a dangerous thing.
Wrong
This is usually quoted by people who would
rather not bother, although it is true of most
politicians. So long as you stick to what you
know and use common sense it is unlikely
you will make the situation any worse.

Once the injured person reaches casualty they are safe.
Wrong
A great deal depends on what you do before the ambulance
arrives. After one hour, the so-called Golden Hour, a
person's fate is more or less sealed. You make the
difference in the equation.

Incredibly dumb things which seemed like a good idea at the time

We all carry ideas on what to do in an emergency. Most of
them come from the movies. It's just as well so few of us
ever saw *Lifeboat* or more people might be hopping to work.

Don't give a casualty anything to eat or drink.
Giving a shipwrecked sailor some sugar after not eating for a
week will cause a massive release of insulin which will take
any remaining sugar out of his blood stream. His reply to 'one

HELP!

lump or two' could be his last. Or if a person is unable to swallow properly, for example after a stroke or head injury, you could choke him.

Don't leave an unconscious or drunk person lying on his back.
Vomit or even his own tongue could block his airway. Jimmy Hendrix was supposed to have moved on to that great rave in the sky this way. After checking his neck for possible fractures, move him into the recovery position.

Don't be afraid to call the emergency services.
If you are not sure whether you are out of your depth, you probably are. Send two people to phone at the same time. It might help if they use different telephones.

Don't use a tourniquet, ever.
Yes, it stops the blood nicely, but once it is released after being on for an hour or two all the gunge in the blood blocks up the kidneys. Still, you can always offer him one of yours. Check you have two kidneys if you've always wanted to have a go wild-west fashion with a neckerchief and a Bowie knife.

Don't ever use your own shirt for bandages. You will never get the stains out. Use someone else's instead.

Don't put yourself in danger.
If it goes wrong, the emergency services have two casualties to deal with. Check your surroundings first for falling rocks, fumes, cars, live electricity or incoming time-share salesmen.

Broken bones

Bones contain blood vessels and nerves, and without them we would all be much shorter and have half-empty cremation urns. A fracture is painful, more so if the broken ends are sticking into flesh. Follow these simple rules:

- Tell the injured person to keep still. Steady and support the limb with your hands.
- Cover any wounds with dressings or clean, non-fluffy material, for example, a cotton shirt. Press as hard as required to stop the bleeding. Bandage the dressing onto the limb.
- If a leg is broken, tie both legs together with a piece of wood or some rolled-up magazines between them. Tie the knees and ankles together first then closer to the broken bone.
- Broken arms or a broken collar bone should be supported by fastening the arm on the affected side to the body.
- Always check that the hands or feet are warm and colour returns after squeezing a nail. If not, loosen the bandages a little. Swelling can tighten bandages, so check every 15 minutes.

Broken spine

A broken neck or spine will not always kill or paralyse you. The guy lifting you up by your lapels probably will. One woman caught her scarf in a car door as it sped off. When the ambulance arrived soon after the relatives explained that the strange thing was she could move her toes until they turned her head the right way round.

Do not move the person unless there is imminent danger within the area. If they must be moved, always support the head and use a number of people to lift in as many places as possible. If available, use a flat piece of wood to carry them on while still supporting their head.

- Reassure the person and tell him not to move. Steady the head with hands on either side of the ears.
- Get helpers to place rolled blankets or coats around his sides to stop him rolling.
- Dial 999 and explain what has happened.
- If you have to wait make a collar from a rolled-up newspaper and cover with a scarf or towel. Wrap it around the neck from the front. Make sure

someone is holding the head firmly as you do so. Check their breathing. Remember this is a collar you are fitting not a tourniquet.

Dislocated joints

Dislocating any joint can damage surrounding nerves, blood vessels, and ligaments. Trying to force the joint back into place can make this ten times worse. Dislocated shoulders are common because it is a relatively lax joint. Horrendous damage can be done when the front row forward decides to 'pop it back in'. Simply support the arm against the front of the body and get them to casualty. Don't give them anything to eat or drink.

Burns

Burns night in casualty means the Guy Fawkes variety not Rabbie. Your chances of survival with 50 per cent burns are almost zero. Even 25 per cent burns can kill if they are not treated quickly.

- Cool the burn area with cold water. This can take ten minutes. Send someone for the ambulance if the burn is severe.
- Remove watches, bracelets or anything which will cause constriction once the flesh begins to swell. This includes shoes and necklaces. Don't remove clothes if they are sticking to the skin.
- Cover the burn area with light non-fluffy material. Don't apply creams or burst any blisters.
- With severe burns there will be a rapid loss of fluid from the blood system with a loss of blood pressure. Lay the person down and raise his legs. This helps keep blood available for the vital organ, as well as the heart, brain, kidneys and lungs.

Choking

It takes surprisingly little to choke a person. Have you ever wondered why you gag when a doctor sticks a teaspoon on the back of your tongue, yet you can eat huge chunks of dead cow and not even hiccup? So have I. Answers on a postcard please. The trick is not to breath in as you swallow. This confuses the epiglottis, a flap which protects the windpipe. Large pieces of dead cow travelling down the wrong pipe will give your complexion a delicate hint of the colour blue.

- Check inside their mouth. If you can see the offending obstruction, pull it out.
- If you can't see it, bend them over and use the flat of your hand to slap them firmly on the back between the shoulder blades five times. A horrible crunching noise means you are enjoying your work far too much.
- If all this fails, go for the Heimlich manoeuvre, which also carries the rather provocative name of the abdominal thrust. This is not what young men consider the normal way of dancing, but instead a highly effective way of causing an explosive release of air up the windpipe.

1   Stand behind your blue patient. Put both arms around their waist and interlock your hands.
2   Pull sharply upwards below the ribs. Note the operative word, 'explosive'. Aim away from your cannelloni, you may never know the difference. Try five times and go back to number one.

Eye injury

Eyes are amazingly tough. Blows from blunt instruments, such as a squash ball, cause extensive damage to the surrounding bone but the eye usually comes out intact. Penetrating injuries are a different matter. Flakes of steel from a chisel struck with a hammer travel at the speed of sound. That's significantly faster than the blink of an eye.

- Lay the injured person on their back and examine the eye. Only irrigate the eye if there is no obvious foreign body stuck to the eye or if there is no open wound.
- Place a loose pad over the eye and bandage.
- Take them to hospital. Avoid stories of the battle of Trafalgar, Nelson and Hardy, especially Hardy.

Heart attacks

Heart disease is the single biggest killer of men, so you are likely to see it happen at some time. Modern drugs can now save most men if they can be kept alive long enough. Recognise what's going on. Central chest pain can move upwards to the throat or arms, usually the left arm. Fear causes the release of adrenaline, which makes the heart beat faster increasing the pain, so talk calmly and reassure. Call for an ambulance as well as the local doctor. If the person normally takes a tablet or oral spray for chest pain, let him do so. Sit him down but don't force him to lie down if he doesn't want to. Give him an aspirin to chew on – it stops any more clots forming in his coronary blood vessels which caused the heart attack. Don't give him anything else to eat or drink.

Cardiac arrest

Simply reading how to perform cardiopulmonary resuscitation (CPR) is like expecting to be able to play a piano after looking at the score for *An American in Paris*. You need to practise before having to do it for real.

Call 999. Check the ABC – Airways, Breathing and Circulation. Shout to see if he responds. Clear the airway by extending the head backwards. Clear the mouth of any debris. Listen for breathing. Check for a pulse at the carotid artery in the neck. If there is no breathing or pulse start CPR.

Lay the person on his back. Tip the head backwards. Pinch his nostrils with one hand while holding the mouth open with the other. Give five strong breaths straight into his mouth. Check his chest is rising each time. If not, make sure the airway is clear; his tongue may have slipped backwards. Give him one good thump in the middle of his chest. Interlace your fingers and place them two-finger breadths up from the middle of the edge of the ribcage. Give him two good thrusts downwards. Keep your arms straight with each thrust. Give two strong breaths into his mouth, as described earlier. Check for a pulse. Alternate 15 chest compressions while counting 'one and two and three' with two breaths into his mouth. You are aiming for about 90 compressions per minute. Maintain this rhythm until help arrives. Get someone else to do either of the two tasks. Swap over if there is a delay in help arriving as it is hard and unpleasant work doing the mouth-to-mouth resuscitation. If you get too light-headed or vomit, get someone else to take over. Time, and keeping the blood circulating, is the essence. Don't mentally whip yourself if he doesn't survive. At least you tried, which is more than many would.

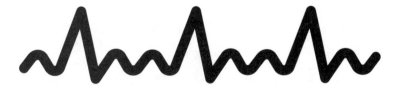

Heavy bleeding

You have got about ten pints of the red stuff in your body. Leaking this blood is never a good idea, particularly from an artery. Lay the person down. Bleeding from a vein is generally slower and simply pressing a cloth against the wound and raising the affected limb above the level of the heart will stop the bleeding Don't believe me? Look at the veins in your hand. Now raise it above your head. Presto! No veins. Arterial bleeds are a different matter. It's hard to miss when it happens. The blood is bright red and comes out in spurts with each heartbeat. Stuff a shirt or cloth against the wound. Press hard.

If you have to leave him, tightly tie a shirt or towel around the pack. Raise their arms and legs to keep the blood pressure up. Some seepage will occur but you will save their life.

Learn the skills

All the first aid voluntary organisations (British Red Cross, St John Ambulance, Order of Malta Ambulance Corp, St Andrew's Ambulance) run courses for beginners. They are the experts and will teach you how to save someone else's life. It is also one of the few legal ways to meet total strangers and kiss them. Really, really kiss them.

Fifteen ways to get the best out of doctors (even if they are male)

A patient once came into casualty and demanded to be seen by a male doctor. As luck would have it I had just delivered a letter so I fitted the bill, as I told him smiling. He didn't smile back, not even a little bit. If being a man can be dangerous, being a man with a male doctor could seriously damage your health. When you next visit your male doctor it is worth remembering that all the statistics true of men are just as true of this one even if he happens to have MB after his name.

Male medics

Even when men do build up enough courage or find the time to visit their doctor, the risk-taking doesn't stop. Medicine is male-dominated. Although the number of women entering general practice now outnumbers men, the ratio of male to female GPs is still 3:1. This has implications for our survival. Doctors are trained to be self-reliant, never to admit a mistake and not to complain in the face of adversity. All the male attitudes towards personal health are just as entrenched in male doctors as they are in any other man. If you attend your doctor with a sore ear, for instance, he is unlikely to say, 'While you're here, I'll just examine your testicles.' Yet there are over 1,600 cases of testicular cancer in the UK each year of which 130 men will die. With early diagnosis few if any of them need to lose their lives, as modern treatment for testicular cancer is highly effective. Women, on the other hand, would generally expect to be advised on cervical and breast cancer and would not think it strange to be shown how to examine their own breasts whatever the original reason for their attendance.

Physician heal thyself

At present male GPs have the dubious distinction of suffering more alcohol-related and stress-related diseases than in any other branch of the medical profession. An alcoholic is now cynically defined as someone who drinks more than their doctor. Suicide is also increasing amongst family doctors and the British Medical Association recently established a confidential stress helpline. It can hardly cope with the demand. Increasing workload and poor morale following the NHS 'reforms' are thought to be the main causes.

To get the best out of a male doctor you need to take all this into consideration. Don't keep him in the dark and don't leave things to chance. Remember, early diagnosis can often make the difference between life and death.

Not mind-readers

Wouldn't it be lovely if you went to your doctor and didn't need to explain just why you happen to be vomiting all over his computer terminal. If only they had a multi-tasking, omnispecies, intergalactic, diagnostic doofer just like Bones in *Star Trek*. A patient once asked me for a second opinion on a suspected flea bite. I waved a ball-point pen with all the different colours over the tiny wound making the appropriate bleep-bleep noises and 'confirmed' the diagnosis. My patient quite rightly gave me a look which reminded me to check my medical insurance. Although everyone rightfully expects an examination from their doctor, most diagnoses are actually made before hands touch flesh. If you approach your physician with the attitude of 'it's my job to know and your job to find out' don't be surprised if you leave with one arm empty for blood tests. Vets and casualty doctors share a common dilemma: they both work out what is wrong with their patients from little or no history. Unless the dog is very clever, a vet cannot even depend upon two woofs for yes, one woof for no. Similarly, the casualty doctor often deals with unconscious patients.

Elementary my dear Watson

Sorting out what is relevant and what is window-dressing can be difficult. Many patients want to tell their doctors every tiny detail, just in case. Information overload confuses the story, impeding decision-making and diagnosis. Why do doctors stick thermometers in your mouth? To check your temperature? Possibly, but this will be a marginally useful by-product. The real reason is that few people, no matter how verbose, can talk with a gob full of mercury and glass. Mercury thermometers are the clinical equivalent of a roll of insulating tape. If your doctor is really after zero decibels, he will also grab your wrist and pointedly count your pulse for a full minute. He only actually needs to do it for 15 seconds and multiply by 4 but during the interval he is looking at your face, hands and chest. Checking your blood pressure is another ploy. He might even tell you the result.

'One hundred and forty over ninety,' he will mutter.

'Is that bad?' you ask.

'Not really,' he answers, with a look on his face that reminds you doctors once considered leeches their best friends.

Doctor Chip

Computers can make a diagnosis, but they cannot decide whether you are telling lies or are simply confused. Doctors check what you are saying against what they find on examination. Imagine attending your doctor with vomiting and a sore gut. After listening to the story for a few minutes he asks you to stick out your tongue and pokes you in the belly a few times. 'Gastroenteritis,' he declares and writes a prescription for a bottle of something which tastes like peppermint chalk mainly because it is chalk flavoured with peppermint. The diagnosis of gastroenteritis is based upon your story, 'the history', and finding nothing serious on examination. But he has checked it out. Skin, for instance, covers the tongue. The normal pink colour is maintained by food scraping off the white surface skin and exposing the pink stuff underneath. If you really were vomiting for the past few days and not eating, your tongue would be white or 'coated'. A bright blue colour simply means you were doing a crossword in the waiting room. A sore gut could possibly be appendicitis. The appendix is an extension of the caecum, part of the large bowel. It is about the length of your little finger. Acute appendicitis is like having a soldering iron waggling about in your belly. A thin internal layer of the abdominal wall, the peritoneum, just hates being touched by soldering irons. When the abdominal wall is pushed down it presses the peritoneum onto the hot appendix. Quickly letting go causes the appendix to wobble and, presto, you hit the ceiling. It's called 'rebound' tenderness and few self-respecting cases of appendicitis would be without it. He simply checked to see if your history fits with his observations. Common illnesses present commonly, so by eliminating anything serious like appendicitis or an ulcer he can allow nature to do the healing.

He who dares usually dies

In 1990 in the UK over 143 million women attended their doctor, more than twice the number of men.

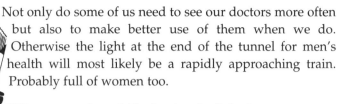

Not only do some of us need to see our doctors more often but also to make better use of them when we do. Otherwise the light at the end of the tunnel for men's health will most likely be a rapidly approaching train. Probably full of women too.

Fifteen ways to get the best out of doctors:

1 **Write down your symptoms before you see your doctor**
It is horribly easy to forget the most important things during the examination. Doctors home in on important clues. When did it start? How did it feel? Did anyone else suffer as well? Did this ever happen before? What have you done about it so far? Are you on any medicines at present?

2 **Respect his professionalism**
Nobody likes a smart ass telling them their job. Turning up with the complete Open University Health and Disease course under your arm may not be conducive to the good doctor/patient relationship. At the same time some doctors can be too paternalistic for modern man.

3 **Ask questions**
If a car mechanic stuck his head into the bonnet of your Porsche, you would most certainly want to know what he intended doing. This doctor is about to lift the bonnet on your body for goodness sake. It is almost as important as your car.

4 **Watch out for over-investigation**
Litigation against doctors is now big business. Defensive medicine can lead to unnecessary tests and investigations. Most x-ray examinations of the painful low back are completely useless. Similarly, isolated cholesterol tests can be misleading. Ask whether the test will really help your diagnosis and treatment.

5 **Avoid asking for night visits unless there is a good reason**
Requests for a home call have quadrupled since 1990. Calling your GP after you have 'suffered' all day at work will antagonise a doctor who thinks personal health should come before convenience. If you put money before the doctor's quality of family life, don't be surprised if you are asked to come to the surgery the following morning.

6 **Don't prevaricate**
If you have a lump on your goolies say so. There are 1,600 cases of testicular cancer each year in the UK. With an average of only two minutes for each consultation there is a real danger of coming out with a prescription for a sore nose if you don't tell your doctor what's wrong.

7 **Health promotion as once decreed by the government is no more**
Now is the time to convince your family doctor to take a serious look at men's health, in particular yours. No screening system exists at present but nothing prevents you from asking for a consultation to examine risk factors. A strong family history of heart disease along with your peccadillo for eating raw blubber and chips might just prompt a blood cholesterol test.

8 **Listen to what he says**
If you don't understand, say so. It helps if they write down the important points. Most people pick up less than half of what their doctor has told them.

9 **Have your prescription explained**
Three items on a script will cost you as much as a half-decent remould. Ask whether you can buy any of them across the counter. Make sure you know what they are all for. Some medicines clash badly with alcohol. Even one pint of beer with the popular antibiotic

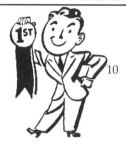

metronidazole (Flagyl) will make you feel very ill. Mixing antidepressants and alcohol can be fatal.

10 **If you want a second opinion say so**
Ask for a consultant appointment by all means but remember you are dealing with a person with feelings and not a computer. Compliment him for his attention first but then explain your deep anxiety.

11 **Flattery will get you anywhere**
Praise is thin on the ground these days. An acknowledgement of a good effort, even if not successful, will be remembered.

12 **Be consistent with all the staff**
Receptionists are not all dragons and practice nurses increasingly influence your treatment. General practice is a team effort and you will get the best out of it by treating all its members with respect. The doctor is not God. The practice manager only lets him think he is.

13 **Be prepared to complain**
If possible see your doctor first and explain what is annoying you. Most complaints against doctors are for rudeness and poor communication, usually as a result of work pressure. Family doctors now have an in-house complaints system. If you are still not satisfied, you can take it to a formal hearing.

14 **Trust your doctor**
There is a difference between trust and blind faith. Your health is a partnership between you and your doctor where you are the majority stakeholder. Despite everything the government has done to the NHS, the majority of people who work in it are still driven by vocation.

15 **Change your GP with caution**
Thousands of people change their doctor each year. Most of them have simply moved house. You do not need to tell your family doctor if you wish to leave their practice. Your new doctor will arrange for all your notes

to be transferred. Like the Doomsday Option in *Dr Strangelove*, changing your doctor should not be done lightly. The whole point of general practice is to build up a personal insight into the health of you and your family. A new doctor has to start from scratch.

Don't be afraid to ask to see your notes. Most doctors now show their patients what they are writing. Unfortunately a doctor's language can be difficult to follow – pharmacists train for four years to be able to understand it. Latin and Greek are still in common usage Worse still, doctors use abbreviations in your notes. Watch out for:

Supratentorial

Conscious thought and automatic bodily functions are located in different parts of the brain separated by a membrane called the tentorium. The upper part looks after personality, memory, writing and speech. Below the tentorium the brain makes sure you are still breathing. If your doctor thinks you are deluding yourself over your symptoms, the real problem lies above the tentorium.

Hysteria

A dangerous diagnosis. Few doctors will be brave enough, or stupid enough, to write this in their notes. It is as good as writing a blank cheque should a patient decide to sue. According to Aristotle, only women can be hysterical. The term derives from hysterus, the womb. He reckoned the symptoms of hysteria were caused by the uterus migrating around the abdomen. Sex and pregnancy were the only cure. Who said men are stupid?

TATT

An abbreviation for Tired All The Time.

TCA SOS

To Call Again if things get worse. Most illnesses are self-limiting. A couple of weeks usually allows nature to sort things out.

RV

Review. Secretaries will automatically arrange a subsequent appointment, subject to you still actually being alive.

PEARLA

Pupils Equal and Reacting to Light and Accommodation. A standard entry on a casualty sheet. It basically means you could still walk and chew gum at the same time, if only your legs were in communication with your inebriated brain.

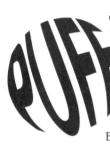

C_2H_5OH

The chemical formula for ethyl alcohol. Often followed in the notes by +++. These are not kisses although you may as well kiss your driving licence goodbye.

RTA

Road Traffic Accident. A combination of RTA and C_2H_5OH in your notes is synonymous with NOB. Now On Bike, or worse. Much, much worse.

FROM

Full Range Of Movement. Usually written after you complain you cannot move your neck after being in an RTA and before seeing a solicitor.

SOB

Short Of Breath. If this comes on after walking in from the waiting room it turns into SOBOE – On Exercise.

AMA/CMA

Against Medical Advice/Contrary Medical Advice. You went home with your neck in a sling.

TTFO

Told to leave the A & E department very abruptly.

FUBAR

Damaged Beyond All Repair: Or words to that effect.

PIP

Pyjama Induced Paralysis. Once those jim-jams go on the power of voluntary movement mysteriously disappears.

DNA

Did Not Attend. You didn't turn up for your appointment.

DNA X 5

Did Not Attend for five arranged appointments.

FU2

Follow-up highly unlikely. Usually follows DNA X 5.

Useful addresses

AIDS helpline (National 24-hour freephone) 0800 567123;
(Northern Ireland) 01232 249268

Alcoholics Anonymous (AA)
General Service Office, PO Box 1, Stonebow House, Stonebow,
York, North Yorks. YO1 2NJ
TEL 01904 644026/7/8/9
  Helplines:
  London: 0171 352 3001; Belfast: 01232 681084;
  Dublin: 003531 4538998

BHAN (Black HIV and AIDS Network)
1st Floor, St Stevens House, 41 Uxbridge Road, London W12 8LH
TEL 0181 749 2828 FAX 0181 746 2898

Body Positive
51B Philbeach Gardens, Earls Court,
London SW5 9EB
TEL 0171 835 1045 FAX 0171 373 5237

British Assocation for Cardiac Rehabilitation
Wellesley House, 117 Wellington Road, Dudley,
West Midlands DY1 1UB
TEL 01384 230222/230601 FAX 01384 254457

British Association of Counselling
1 Regent Place, Rugby CV21 2PJ
TEL 01788 578328

British Association of Sexual and Marital Therapy
PO Box 62, Sheffield S40 1UU

British Colostomy Association
15 Station Road, Reading, Berks RG1 1LG
TEL 01189 391537 FAX 01189 569095

British Digestive Foundation
3 St Andrew's Place, London NW1 4LB
TEL 0171 486 0341 FAX 0171 224 2012

British Heart Foundation
14 Fitzhardinge Street, London W1H 4DH
TEL 0171 935 0185 FAX 0171 486 5820

British Hernia Centre
87 Waterford Way, London NW4 4RS
TEL 0181 201 7000 FAX 0181 202 6714

British Red Cross
9 Grosvenor Crescent, London SW1X 7EJ
TEL 0171 235 5454 FAX 0171 245 6315

> **Northern Ireland headquarters**
> 87 University Street, Belfast BT7 1HP
> TEL 01232 246400 FAX 01232 326102

Brook Advisory Clinics
233 Tottenham Court Road, London W1P 9AE
TEL 0171 323 1522

> **Northern Ireland headquarters**
> 29A North Street, Belfast BT1 1NA
> TEL 01232 328866 FAX 01232 235735

Colon Health
27 Warwick Avenue, London W9 2PS
TEL 0171 289 7000 FAX 0171 286 1592

Continence Helpline
2 Doughty Street, London W21N 2PH
TEL 0191 2130050

Coronary Prevention Group
42 Store Street, London WC1E 7DB
TEL 0171 580 1070 FAX 0171 436 6220

Dublin AIDS Alliance
53 Parnell Square, Dublin 1
Helpline 003531 8724277

Family Planning Association
2–12 Pentonville Road, London N1 9FP
TEL 0171 837 5432 FAX 0171 837 3026

Family Planning Association (NI)
113 University Street, Belfast BT7 1HP
TEL 01232 325488 FAX 01232 312212

Health Education Authority
Hamilton House, Mabledon Place, London WC1H 9TX
TEL 0171 383 3833 FAX 0171 387 0550

Hearing Concern (British Association of the Hard of Hearing)
7–11 Armstrong Road, London W3 7JL
TEL 0181 743 1110 FAX 0181 742 9043

Heart, Chest and Stroke Association
21 Dublin Road, Belfast BT2 7FJ
TEL 01232 320184 FAX 01232 333487

Terrence Higgins Trust
52–54 Gray's Inn Road, London WC1X 8JU
Helpline 0171 242 1010 (12 noon to 10 PM)

Impotence Information Centre
PO Box 1130, London W3 0BB

International Stress Management Association UK
South Bank University, LPSS, 103 Borough Road, London SE1 0AA
TEL 01992 633100

Irish Association for Cardiac Rehabilitation
Beaumont Hospital, Dublin 1
TEL 003531 8377755 (EX 2816)

McCormack Group
(for information on TSE [testicular self-examination])
Church House, Church Square,
Leighton Buzzard, Beds LU7 7AE
TEL 01525 851313   FAX 01525 851314

Manic Depression Fellowship
8–10 High Street, Kingston upon Thames, Surrey KT1 1EY
TEL 0181 974 6550 FAX 0181 974 6600

Mental Health Association
Mensana House, 6 Adelaide Street,
Dun Laoghaire, County Dublin
TEL 003531 2841166 FAX 003531 2841736

MIND
(National Association for Mental Health)
Granta House, 15–19 Broadway, Stratford, London E15 4BQ
TEL 0181 519 2122 FAX 0181 522 1725

Northern Ireland headquarters
80 University Street, Belfast BT7 1HE
TEL 01232 328474 FAX 01232 234940

Prostate Association
Stanley House, 22 Paradise Street, Rugby CV21 3SZ
TEL 01788 543176

QUIT
Victory House, 170 Tottenham Court Road, London W1P 0HA
Smokers' quitline: 0171 487 3000
(MON to FRI 1 PM to 9 PM; SAT to SUN 1 PM to 5 PM)

Relate Marriage Guidance
Herbert Gray College, Little Church Street, Rugby CV21 3AP
TEL 01788 573241 FAX 01788 535007

Northern Ireland headquarters
76 Dublin Road, Belfast BT2 7HP
TEL 01232 323454 FAX 01232 315298

St John Ambulance
1 Grosvenor Crescent, London SW1X 7ES
TEL 0171 235 5231 FAX 0171 235 0796

Northern Ireland headquarters
Erne, Knockbracken Health Care Park,
Saintfield Road, Belfast BT8 8RA
TEL 01232 799393 FAX 01232 793303

Republic of Ireland headquarters
Lumsden House, 29 Upper Leeson Street, Dublin 4
TEL 003531 6688077

Samaritans
General Office, 10 The Grove, Slough, Berks SL1 1QP
TEL 01753 532713 FAX 01753 775787

Northern Ireland headquarters
5 Wellesley Avenue, Belfast BT9 6DG
TEL 01232 664422 FAX 01232 683962

Republic of Ireland headquarters
112 Marlborough Street, Dublin 1
TEL 003531 8727700

Index